AGING AND HEALTH

SOME OTHER VOLUMES IN THE
SAGE FOCUS EDITIONS

AGING AND HEALTH

Perspectives on Gender, Race, Ethnicity, and Class

Edited by
Kyriakos S. Markides

SAGE PUBLICATIONS
The Publishers of Professional Social Science
Newbury Park   London   New Delhi

Copyright © 1989 by Sage Publications, Inc.

For information address:

SAGE Publications, Inc.
2111 West Hillcrest Drive
Newbury Park, California 91320

SAGE Publications Ltd.
28 Banner Street
London EC1Y 8QE
England

SAGE Publications India Pvt. Ltd.
M-32 Market
Greater Kailash I
New Delhi 110 048 India

Printed in the United States of America

Library of Congress Cataloging-in-Publication Data

Main entry under title:

Aging and health.

    (Sage focus editions ; v. 104)
    Bibliography: p.
    1. Aged—Health and hygiene—United States.
2. Aging—United States. I. Markides, Kyriakos S.
Includes index
RA564.8.A389   1989   362.1'9897'00973   88–35932
ISBN 0–8039–3206–5
ISBN 0–8039–3207–3 (pbk.)

FIRST PRINTING 1989

Contents

Preface

Even though social gerontology has exhibited phenomenal growth in recent decades, much of the field has had a definite social psychological focus aimed at describing "successful" aging, which has been typically operationalized in terms of such concepts as life satisfaction, morale, and mental health. Efforts at uncovering predictors of successful aging have been met with modest results. By far the most important predictor has been a person's health, usually operationalized in terms of self-ratings given by the elderly.

In recent years, social gerontologists have shown increased interest in studying predictors of the health of older people. Health is increasingly becoming a key concern, and approaches to its study are becoming more sophisticated. It is becoming apparent that relying on people's global definitions of their health provides highly partial information on a complex subject, information that gives few guidelines to social and health policy aimed at improving the health status of the elderly.

A welcome change has been the recent interest of epidemiologists in studying the health of older people. Epidemiologists have traditionally restricted their studies to persons under 65. This was probably a reflection of society's generally ageist attitudes, which viewed studies of the prevalence (or incidence) of disease or disability in older people as less fruitful than similar studies of younger people. At the same time, the few studies that existed revealed that traditional risk factors for major diseases (and mortality from them) were not as predictive among older people as was the case with younger people.

However, recent demographic, political, and social changes have made it desirable to apply epidemiologic approaches to the study of older people. The numbers of older people are rising faster than anticipated just five or ten years ago, primarily because of recent improvements in life expectancy at older ages. It is also becoming apparent that increased survival is accompanied by increased concentration of health problems and disability in advanced old age. The short-term outlook is for an increasing societal burden both in terms of financing needed medical care and in terms of the rising dependency of older people on younger generations within the family.

This book's aim is to gather available data and literature on aging and health and organize them into various chapters focusing on particular groups within the American population. By doing so, we hope to both facilitate and stimulate research on aging and health that goes beyond the collection and analysis of relatively simple data based on self-reports. In particular, large-scale social epidemiologic approaches to the health of older people can benefit a great deal by the information.

The chapters that follow focus on gender, class, and race/ethnic differences in health, and how these change with aging. It is hoped that the data and analyses presented will provide a modest contribution to the understanding of how social structural variables influence the health of people as they get older.

This book owes a great deal to Terry Hendrix from Sage Publications, whose interest and encouragement throughout have been invaluable. Ann Winkler has read several of the chapters and has made useful comments and suggestions. Finally, I acknowledge Kandy Burke's expert typing and good sense of humor, paricularly during the preparation of the final manuscript while Hurricane Gilbert was threatening the Gulf of Mexico coast.

—Kyriakos S. Markides

CHAPTER 1

Aging, Gender, Race/Ethnicity, Class, and Health

A Conceptual Overview

KYRIAKOS S. MARKIDES

Social gerontologists have always been interested in the health of populations and individuals, but few studies they conducted over the years have been systematic enough to make significant contributions to knowledge about how social, psychological, and cultural factors influence people's health as they age. Rather, they have concentrated their efforts, both empirical and conceptual, on understanding how health and other factors influence older people's "successful adjustment" to aging and old age (Maddox and Wiley, 1976). Successful adjustment has been variously operationalized using broadly defined measures of life satisfaction, morale, psychological well-being, and mental health.

Systematic understanding of health itself as an important outcome was left to demographers and epidemiologists. Demographers have traditionally concentrated on studying mortality rates through the use of life tables and related techniques. Much of this work has been mathematical in nature and descriptive in the sense of computing and presenting mortality rates and life expectancy figures for various ages. Because of data limitations and the need for large samples, attention to other factors has been limited. Although changes are underway, life tables have routinely been published only by sex and by race. Needless to say, the contributions of demographic analysis to our understanding of the health of populations have been invaluable.

Epidemiologists, on the other hand, have employed a variety of techniques to study the health of populations. Large-scale community surveys have been employed to estimate the incidence and prevalence of a variety of diseases as well as to predict mortality from these diseases. A variety of predictors ("risk factors") have been introduced to explain health outcomes, including biological (e.g., cholesterol levels), social (e.g., social class), psychological (Type A behavior pattern), and behavioral (e.g., smoking). A "taken-for-granted" risk factor always to be controlled in studies of chronic disease prevalence and incidence, as well as mortality from these diseases, has been chronological age. After all, as a quick glance at a life table would reveal, age bears a fairly linear and strong association with mortality. It is also strongly related to the incidence of major chronic diseases.

Most epidemiologic studies, however, have traditionally limited themselves to middle-aged and younger subjects and typically have not included older people. This practice may well reflect "ageist" attitudes; it was not uncommon to feel, for example, that knowledge about what predicts the health of older people was less valuable because they had fewer productive years left or because it might be too late to make much difference in their longevity. There was also a realization that traditional risk factors did not predict as well in old age.

In recent years we have witnessed new large-scale epidemiologic studies of the health of older people, funded primarily by the National Institute on Aging. The greatest challenge for these studies is the success-ful search for new and nontraditional risk factors. This task is further complicated by the presence of multiple conditions in older people, as well as by recent increases in the life expectancy at advanced ages.

As we near the end of the twentieth century, it is becoming increas-ingly evident that aging is everybody's business and the health of older people is a key concern of scholars from a variety of disciplines. No doubt, the aging of the population has a great deal to do with this interest. However, gerontologists can take a great deal of pride in the increasing societal awareness of the social, psychological, and economic problems of modern society's elderly. This increased aware-ness is, in turn, permitting the allocation of resources for addressing these problems and for generating a better understanding of the aging process.

We are indeed becoming more sophisticated in our approaches to understanding the aging process and its concomitants. We are also seeing that our research is becoming increasingly interdisciplinary. Sociologists, psychologists, epidemiologists, biologists, physicians, and others are learning from each other and are contributing to each other's understanding of what happens to the health of people as they get older.

AGE AND HEALTH

As mentioned earlier, perhaps the most established association with health has been that of chronological age. It has been commonly assumed that aging is accompanied by a fairly progressive, although variable, deterioration of physical health. In addition to evidence on mortality rates, cross-sectional data using a variety of measures of health have consistently supported the association between age and health. It is also true that many health differences observed in cross-sectional studies are to some extent the result of cohort or generational influences because of steady improvements of the population's health. This generalization, however, must be made with caution because it is not clear that the health of populations has improved at all ages. There is, for example, some evidence that we are living longer but with more disability in the older years (Verbrugge, 1984).

The argument that increased survival might be associated with more disability concentrated in late middle age and old age runs counter to the "compression of morbidity" perspective that has been so popular and so influential during the 1980s (Fries, 1980). According to this perspective, because of better health practices, better care, and other factors, modern society is increasingly postponing illness and disability until later in life. Because the life span is "fixed" around ages 85 to 90, we are rapidly approaching the upper biological limits. This would translate into longer lives free of disability and a shorter period of disability followed by a quicker death for most people. This compression of morbidity is likely to reduce the demand for medical care and result in savings of health care dollars.

Needless to say, this optimistic scenario has met with a great deal of controversy and has been questioned by scholars from a variety of disciplines. Scholars who questioned the assumptions of the compression of morbidity thesis have pointed to evidence arguing that the opposite is taking place (see, for example, Myers & Manton, 1983; Schneider & Brody, 1983). Thus, we are seeing increased concentration of health problems in old age and a higher demand on health care resources.

Verbrugge's (1984) findings are consistent with greater disability in old age as is the general argument that we are witnessing lower levels of "selective survival" as people are kept alive longer by better health care and better health practices (Markides & Machalek, 1984). The picture of the association between aging and health is becoming further complicated by an unexpected rise in the life expectancy of people who are already old. Verbrugge documents these trends in her chapter in this volume (see also Crimmins, 1984; Rosenwaike, 1985).

Trends in the association between age and mortality (or other health indicators) make clear that the relationship between age and health is variable and subject to change. There is, however, a biological imperative that suggests that, other things equal, there are biological factors making progressive declines in health as people get older.

Although age is typically treated as a biological variable in studies of the health of populations, gerontologists have argued for decades that age is also a sociological variable. Prominent in this literature has been the work of Matilda Riley (1972, 1976, 1985), which has proposed an age stratification perspective. Thus, variation in the age-related decline in health is modified by social and environmental factors concomitant with aging. Age stratification formulations that owe a great deal to Riley's pioneer work have more recently treated age as another stratification factor to be treated as another source of inequality much like class, race/ethnicity, and gender (see, for example, Bengtson, 1979).

If age is to be treated as a source of inequality, it follows that it would result in differentials in power, prestige, and life chances, and scholars have outlined over the years such differences between age groups (Dowd, 1980; Streib, 1985). Moreover, if age is a source of inequality, it should influence people's health over and above biology. Unfortunately, little research has been directly aimed at exploring this hypothesis.

As we will see below, the sociological significance of age and health has received some attention by scholars in the minority aging literature who have argued that minority status should magnify the negative effects of aging (Dowd & Bengtson, 1978; Jackson, 1985; Markides, 1983; Varghese & Medinger, 1979). Aging and old age can be seen as a burden in modern society because they are devalued. Thus aging is stressful and should take its toll on health. Moreover, older people have fewer resources for coping with stress, and their health is accordingly affected.

This social stress interpretation of the effects of aging on health has been refined in more recent years by scholars working in the area of life course transitions (George, 1980; House, 1983; Markides & Cooper, 1989). With regard to older people, most research has concentrated on single major transitions, such as retirement, widowhood and institutionalization. Although we have assumed that these major transitions are stressful, we have failed to document that they have adverse outcomes on people's health. Review of the evidence in ten industrialized societies has failed to show any negative effects of retirement (Markides & Cooper, 1987; see also Ekerdt et al., 1983). With regard to widowhood, the evidence is at best unclear (Ferraro, 1989) as it is with respect to institutionalization (Tobin, 1989) and residential relocation (Baglioni, 1989).

Another approach to examining the stress potentially entailed in life course transitions has been the summation of multiple events (transitions) within a specified period of time. Unfortunately, the life events research has generally ignored older people. Moreover, there are numerous methodological problems in developing life events measures comparable across age groups (Chiriboga, 1989).

Research on life course transitions has recently focused on distinguishing between normative transitions that are expected or sheduled, such as retirement at age 65, and unscheduled or unexpected transitions, such as widowhood in young adulthood (House, 1983; Pearlin & Radabaugh, 1980). In addition, Pearlin and Radabaugh (1980) have emphasized the importance of "role strains" that are durable problems and conflicts that do not involve transitions. Persistent marital problems, for example, may entail more stress than divorce itself.

Although ways of studying how life course transitions, events, and role strains influence people's health are developing, much remains to be done with regard to how older people are differently influenced than younger people. Yet this is an evolving area of considerable promise since it brings together the conceptual work of social scientists with the methodological rigor of epidemiologists.

GENDER, AGING, AND HEALTH

Another key variable in health research has been sex or gender. As Verbrugge suggests in this book, sex, like age, is fundamentally a biological variable. Yet it is also a social variable, more appropriately labeled gender. As such, both biological and psychosocial factors are involved in explaining sex and gender differentials in the health of people. The added dimension that must be tackled simultaneously, as Verbrugge does, is how aging modifies the association between sex or gender and health. This is an area where a considerable amount of work has been conducted over the years. Both regional studies and national data have been available for a long time to answer the critical questions asked by this book. Women do indeed live considerably longer than men and have done so for a long time. Moreover, the gender gap in life expectancy at birth has increased throughout the twentieth century, although it has declined a bit in the 1980s. The gender gap in life expectancy is also considerably narrower in old age.

Why do women live longer than men? According to Verbrugge, both biological (genetic or hormonal) and psychosocial factors, such as men's smoking more, consuming more alcohol, and being prone to more violent and risky behavior, are involved. These factors translate into higher life expectancy for women at every age. These differences result from the greater prevalence of major chronic diseases, such as cardiovascular diseases and malignant neoplasms. On the other hand, the evidence amassed by Verbrugge suggests that women of all ages suffer more from nonfatal conditions, particularly arthritis. Women also suffer more from a variety of minor illnesses and limitations in activities of daily life, with the gender gap in the latter increasing with age.

Despite the availability of high quality data, there remains a great deal of mystery about gender differences in health and how these are modified with age. The National Institute on Aging, for example, has undertaken a major funding initiative aimed at explaining the male-female gap in life expectancy.

CLASS, AGING, AND HEALTH

Class differs from age and gender in that it has no direct biological basis. It is a social structural variable whose influence on health can be understood within a social stratification perspective. People are born, grow up, and grow old in different socioeconomic strata, which influence their life chances as well as their health. The link between socioeconomic status and health has been observed for a long time and has become an established premise in medical sociology and social epidemiology (Kaplan, Haan, Syme, Minkler, & Winkleby, 1987).

Reasons for the association between socioeconomic status and health are many and include the stresses associated with poverty, absence of resources for dealing with stress, poor access to health care, as well as health practices and behaviors associated with poor health among lower status groups.

There is overwhelming evidence that poor people do not live as long and that they suffer disproportionately from major diseases, such as heart disease, cancer, diabetes and hypertension. They also experience decreased survival from cancer and from a heart attack (Kaplan et al., 1987). Significant class associations with other diseases or illnesses are too numerous to mention.

Despite its importance to people's health, it is surprising how little attention has been given to class and socioeconomic status in recent years. There is, perhaps, the assumption that the association has been established over the years so that our attention needs to be directed to how other factors influence health. As Longino, Warheit, and Green point out in this book, another factor is the absence of mortality data by class. As we saw earlier, life tables are routinely published only by gender and race and not by social class. However, national data from health surveys are increasingly becoming tabulated by class, and epidemiologic studies routinely collect information on class and other socioeconomic status variables. Yet, even though epidemiologists have elevated socioeconomic position to the status of an established "risk factor," Kaplan et al. (1987) wondered why health promotion and disease prevention programs pay so little attention to it. One possible reason, they felt, is the feeling that it is virtually impossible to change people's socioeconomic status through conventional approaches to health promotion.

Gerontologists are also guilty of ignoring social class in their study of the health of older people, as Longino, Warheit, and Green demonstrate. The critical question posed in their study is the extent to which socioeconomic status differences in the middle or younger years of life are carried over into old age. They find that expected socioeconomic status differences are observed in old age, but they are not as great as might be anticipated. They also note that the relationship is complex and must be understood in a dynamic context since aging (survival), class, and health are themselves constantly changing. Longino, Warheit, and Green feel that their analysis is only beginning and more remains to be done to isolate the relationship between social class and the health of the elderly from the effect of other variables.

RACE/ETHNICITY, AGING, AND HEALTH

The importance of social class is frequently emphasized by scholars in the race/ethnicity literature who often point out that the effects of race/ethnicity on health (or other variables) need to be understood independently of the effects of social class (Jackson, 1985; Markides & Mindel, 1987). Despite such cautions, however, many studies evaluate the influence of race/ethnicity without special attention to class. As previously discussed, for example, demographic analyses of life table data are conducted by race/ethnicity but are not typically available separately by social class.

In this volume we give attention to the health of America's three major disadvantaged ethnic groups: blacks, Hispanics, and American Indians. Jackson and Perry review the evidence on blacks; Markides, Coreil, and Rogers limit their attention to southwestern Hispanics, most of whom are Mexican Americans; finally, Kunitz and Levy focus on only one major American Indian group, the Navajos, primarily because of the relative lack of data on other groups.

Of the three groups, considerably more attention has been given to blacks. There are national data on the mortality situation of blacks, and the National Center of Health Statistics routinely publishes life tables displaying their mortality rates and how they compare with the rates of whites (see Jackson & Perry, Chapter 4). National mortality data are not available for Hispanics, and Markides, Coreil, and Rogers rely on data from specific states, particularly from Texas and California where most southwestern Hispanics live. No national data are available on American Indians. Yet the study by Kunitz and Levy on the Navajo Nation has generated a wealth of information on the health of elderly Navajos. As is well-known, data on ethnic groups are characterized by definitional problems as well as by problems of coverage.

Jackson and Perry amass a great deal of information on the mortality and health of middle-aged and older blacks. They note the well-known, wide differences in health status between blacks and whites, and they show them to exist with a wide variety of health indicators. They also note and discuss the existence of racial mortality crossovers involving the crossing of the black and white mortality curves in old age. Although the reality of the racial mortality crossover was questioned when it was first discovered because of age misreporting and other errors in the data, adjustments for such errors failed to eliminate the crossover (Kitagawa & Hauser, 1973; Rives, 1977). The work of

Manton and his colleagues (Manton, Poss, & Wing, 1979; Manton & Stallard, 1981) and more recent longitudinal data (Wing, Manton, Stallard, Homes, & Tyroler, 1985) have strongly suggested that the racial mortality crossover is indeed real and probably results from high early mortality, which removes less hardy blacks before they reach advanced old age so that the group of surviving blacks contains a higher proportion of robust persons than the group of surviving whites. This kind of "selective survival" explanation (see Markides & Machalek, 1984) is also discussed by Jackson and Perry in their chapter. These authors point out that, regardless of whether one believes in the existence of black/white mortality crossover, recent data show that it has been pushed upward from age 75 to around age 85 and over. This rise in the crossover is consistent with the selective survival thesis advanced by Markides and Machalek (1984), who predicted such a rise as mortality rates of blacks in middle and early old age decline.

Given the mechanisms thought to produce the black/white mortality crossover, one would expect to find it in other pairs of advantaged and disadvantaged populations. Kunitz and Levy provide evidence that a crossover also exists among Navajos and non-Navajos. Earlier National Center for Health Statistics (1980) data showed this to be the case for other native Americans and whites. A similar crossover is not evident in the data on Hispanics presented by Markides, Coreil, and Rogers. Yet these authors show (see also Markides & Coreil, 1986) that the overall mortality situation of southwestern Hispanics is not substantially different from that of other whites, so that one would not predict the existence of a Hispanic/other white crossover in old age.

Markides, Coreil, and Rogers review a great deal of evidence bearing on the relative advantage of southwestern Hispanics in relation to blacks. They show that traditionally Hispanics, particularly men, have been protected from major diseases such as heart disease, stroke, and cancer, although this situation appears to be changing. Hispanics, however, experience more diabetes as do Navajos and other American Indian groups. Hispanics and Navajos also have higher accident rates and rates of infectious and parasitic diseases. Navajos are similar to Hispanics in that they too appear to be protected from major cardiovascular diseases and cancer. Kunitz and Levy propose that high early mortality from accidents might be responsible for these low rates among Navajos, since one could make the case that persons dying early from accidents would be more likely to develop cardiovascular diseases had they lived longer than persons who do not die of accidents. The same argument with regard to overall American Indian mortality was also made by Markides and Machalek (1984). Both papers, however, recognize the tentativeness of this argument because of the absence of adequate data on the characteristics of accident victims.

CONCLUSION

The chapters in this book present a great deal of evidence of differences in health by gender, class, and race/ethnicity. Data are by far superior with regard to gender differences and differences between blacks and whites. All five chapters also present evidence that group differences observed in middle age are not as pronounced in old age, and in some cases reverse themselves. Narrowing of differences is particularly pronounced between blacks and whites and between Navajos and whites. With respect to class differences, the evidence is not clear because of the relative lack of mortality and health data by class across the life cycle. Gender differences also appear to decline but do not reverse themselves. Finally, we have no convincing evidence that Hispanic to other white differences decline consistently, and mortality rates do not reverse themselves in old age.

The evidence accumulated in this volume gives credence to the selective survival thesis advanced earlier (Markides & Machalek, 1984). More specifically, disadvantaged high mortality populations appear to experience a greater amount of removal of the least robust persons before old age, so that the surviving elderly in such populations might include a relatively high rate of hardy persons. Extreme situations produce mortality crossovers, as evident among blacks and Navajos, as well as other American Indian populations. The lack of a crossover between the mortality curves of men and women despite wide mortality differences in middle and early old age appears to be an anomaly. Yet as Manton and Stallard (1981) have suggested, crossovers are primarily produced by differential environmental pressures in populations that are initially similar with regard to their genetic endowment for longevity. Based on the available evidence, men and women are not similarly endowed genetically. However, because the mortality gap is partially the result of behavioral and social factors, a narrowing of mortality and health differences between men and women is apparent at advanced ages. And, as Verbrugge illustrates, although the mortality curves of men and women do not cross in old age, there is a high concentration of illness and disability among very old women.

The narrowing of health differences between the groups covered in this volume can finally shed some light on the apparent decline in the predictive importance of social and psychological factors with respect to health and mortality as we move from middle to old age (Branch & Jette, 1984; Riegel, Riegel, and Meyer, 1967). If a disproportionate number of people in certain groups (e.g., blacks, smokers, less intelligent persons) die early, it would be expected that group membership would not be as predictive of mortality and health in the later years. The currently funded, large-scale epidemiologic investigations in the area of aging are likely to shed further light on this matter and might very well produce alternative predictors. We hope that this book is a modest contribution to the emerging literature aimed at understanding the relationship between psychosocial variables and health as people grow old.

REFERENCES

Baglioni, A. J. (1989). Residential relocation and health among the elderly. In K. S. Markides & C. L. Cooper (Eds.), *Aging, stress and health: Social, psychological, and epidemiologic perspectives* (pp. 117-135). Chichester and New York: John Wiley.

Bengtson, V. L. (1979). Ethnicity and aging: Problems and issues in current social science inquiry. In D. E. Gelfand & A. J. Kutzik (Eds.), *Ethnicity and aging: Theory, research and policy* (pp. 9-31). New York: Springer.

Branch, L. G., & Jette, A. M. (1984). Personal health practices and mortality among the elderly. *American Journal of Public Health, 74*, 1126-1129.

Chiriboga, D. A. (1989). The measurement of stress exposure in late life. In K. S. Markides & C. L. Cooper (Eds.), *Aging, stress and health: Social, psychological, and epidemiologic perspectives* (pp. 13-40). Chichester and New York: John Wiley.

Crimmins, E. M. (1984). Life expectancy and the older population. *Research on Aging, 6*, 490-514.

Dowd, J. J. (1980). *Stratification among the aged.* Monterey, CA: Brooks/Cole.

Dowd, J. J., & Bengtson, V. L. (1978). Aging in minority populations: An examination of the double jeopardy hypothesis. *Journal of Gerontology, 33*, 427-436.

Ekerdt, D. J., Baden, L., Bosse, R., & Dibbs, E. (1983). The effect of retirement on physical health. *American Journal of Public Health, 73*, 779-783.

Ferraro, K. (1989). Widowhood and health. In K. S. Markides & C. L. Cooper (Eds.), *Aging, stress and health: Social, psychological, and epidemiologic perspectives.* Chichester and New York: John Wiley.

Fries, J. F. (1980). Aging, natural death and the compression of morbidity. *New England Journal of Medicine, 303*, 130-135.

George, L. K. (1980). *Role transitions in late life.* Belmont, CA: Brooks/Cole.

House, J. S. (1983). Age, psychosocial stress, and health. In M. W. Riley, B. B. Hess, & K. Bond (Eds.), *Aging in society: Selected reviews of recent research* (pp. 175-197). Hillsdale, NJ: Lawrence Erlbaum.

Jackson, J. J. (1985). Race, national origin, ethnicity, and aging. In R. H. Binstock & E. Shanas (Eds.), *Handbook of aging and the social sciences* (2nd ed.) (pp. 264-303). New York: Van Nostrand Reinhold.

Kaplan, G. A., Haan, M. N., Syme, S. L., Minkler, M., & Winkleby, M. (1987). Socioeconomic status and health. In R. W. Amler & H. B. Dull (Eds.), *Closing the gap: The burden of unnecessary illness* (pp. 125-129). New York: Oxford University Press.

Kitagawa, E. M., & Hauser, P. M. (1973). *Differential mortality in the United States: A study in socio-economic epidemiology.* Cambridge, MA: Harvard University Press.

Maddox, G. L., & Wiley, J. (1976). Scope, concepts and methods in the study of aging. In R. H. Binstock & E. Shanas (Eds.), *Handbook of aging and the social sciences* (pp. 3-34). New York: Van Nostrand Reinhold.

Manton, K. G., Poss, S. S., & Wing, S. (1979). The black/white mortality crossover: Investigation from the perspective of the components of aging. *The Gerontologist, 19*, 291-300.

Manton, K. G., & Stallard, E. (1981). Methods for evaluating the heterogeneity of aging processes in human populations using vital statistics data: Explaining the black/white mortality crossover by a model of mortality selection. *Human Biology, 53*, 47-67.

Markides, K. S. (1983). Minority aging. In M. W. Riley, B. B. Hess, & K. Bond (Eds.), *Aging in society: Selected reviews of recent research* (pp. 115-137). Hillsdale, NJ: Lawrence Erlbaum.

Markides, K. S., & Cooper, C. L. (Eds.). (1987). *Retirement in industrialized societies: Social, psychological and health factors.* Chichester and New York: John Wiley.

Markides, K. S., & Cooper, C. L. (Eds.). (1989). *Aging, stress and health: Social, psychological and epidemiologic perspectives.* Chichester and New York: John Wiley.

Markides, K. S., & Coreil, J. (1986). The health of Southwestern Hispanics: An epidemiologic paradox. *Public Health Reports, 101*, 253-265.

Markides, K. S., & Machalek, R. (1984). Selective survival, aging and society. *Archives of Gerontology and Geriatrics, 3*, 207-222.

Markides, K. S., & Mindel, C. H. (1987). *Aging and ethnicity.* Newbury Park, CA: Sage.

Myers, G. C., & Manton, K. G. (1983). Recent changes in the U. S. age at death distribution: Further observations. *The Gerontologist, 24*, 572-575.

National Center for Health Statistics. (1980). *Health, United States—1979.* Public Health Service, Washington, DC: U. S. Government Printing Office.

Pearlin, L., & Radabaugh, C. (1980). Age and stress: Perspectives and problems. In H. McCubbin (Ed.), *Family, stress, coping and social support.* New York: Springer.

Riegel, K. F., Riegel, R. M., & Meyer, G. A. (1967). A study of dropout rates in longitudinal research on aging and the prediction of death. *Journal of Personality and Social Psychology, 5*, 342-348.

Riley, M. W. (1976). Age strata in social systems. In R. H. Binstock & E. Shanas (Eds.), *Handbook of aging and the social sciences* (pp. 189-217). New York: Van Nostrand Reinhold.

Riley, M. W. (1985). Age strata in social systems. In R. H. Binstock & E. Shanas (Eds.), *Handbook of aging and the social sciences* (2nd ed.) (pp. 369-403). New York: Van Nostrand Reinhold.

Riley, M. W., Johnson, M., & Foner, A. (1972). *Aging and society: Vol. III. A sociology of age stratification.* New York: Russell Sage.

Rives, N. W. (1977). The effects of census errors on life table estimates of black mortality. *Public Health Briefs, 67,* 867-868.

Rosenwaike, T. (1985). *The extreme aged in America.* Westport, CT: Greenwood.

Schneider, E. L., & Brody, J. A. (1983). Aging, natural death and the compression of morbidity: Another view. *New England Journal of Medicine, 309,* 854-855.

Streib, G. F. (1985). Social stratification and aging. In R. H. Binstock & E. Shanas (Eds.), *Handbook of aging and the social sciences* (2nd ed.) (pp. 339-368). New York: Van Nostrand Reinhold.

Tobin, S. S. (1989). Institutionalization and health among the elderly. In K. S. Markides & C. L. Cooper (Eds.), *Aging, stress and health: Social, psychological, and epidemiologic perspectives* (pp. 137-161). Chichester and New York: John Wiley.

Varghese, R., & Medinger, F. (1979). Fatalism in response to stress among the minority aged. In D. E. Gelfand & A. J. Kutzik (Eds.), *Ethnicity and aging* (pp. 96-116). New York: Springer.

Verbrugge, L. M. (1984). Longer life but worsening health? Trends in the health and mortality of middle-aged and older persons. *Milbank Memorial Fund Quarterly/Health and Society, 62,* 475-519.

Wing, S., Manton, K. G., Stallard, E. C., Hames, C. G., & Tyroler, H. A. (1985). The black/white mortality crossover: Investigation in a community-based study. *The Journal of Gerontology, 40,* 78-84.

CHAPTER 2

Gender, Aging, and Health

LOIS M. VERBRUGGE

GENDER, AGING, AND HEALTH

They are an odd pair, the two central demographic characteristics: one (sex) is constant across an individual's life, the other (age), perpetually dynamic. One is the bedrock on which gender identity is built. The other is the stream that encourages and forces behavioral change over time. Birth is the official starting point for each from society's stance: sex is noted, and age starts counting.

Both sex and age are fundamentally biological, yet they become densely social—as gender and aging—as a person lives. Gender penetrates and fashions sex. Becoming a child, a youth, and then an adult is a social process woven through biological age. Whether overtly or covertly, sex and age are involved in role training and rewards, the formation and maintenance of close social ties, productive activities at home and elsewhere, and encounters with health risks and their physical and mental outcomes. They are never really separable in social life.

AUTHOR'S NOTE: Preparation of this article was facilitated by a Special Emphasis Research Career Award (KO1 AG00394) from the National Institute on Aging. The author thanks various staff of the National Center for Health Statistics for providing unpublished data for a number of tables (Kate Prager, for selected 1955 mortality data on file and for prepublication 1985 mortality rates by age-sex-cause; Susan Jack, for 1983-85 National Health Interview Survey (NHIS) prevalence rates by age-sex-condition; Peter Ries, for 1979 and 1980 NHIS activity limitation data by age-sex-condition; Gary Collins, for 1986 NHIS self-reported health data by age-sex; Esther Hing, for selected 1985 National Nursing Home Survey estimates).

This article is a gift posthumous to the author's father who died of cancer of bone marrow in 1985, and a gift actual to her mother who copes daily with osteoarthritis.

It is a person's age-sex category, not just age and not just sex, that inspires particular social attitudes and confers certain demands. Together, these two features carry people across their life course, for better or worse in health and social standing.

This chapter is about a key feature of life: physical health and how the entwining of gender and aging leads to different health experiences for middle-aged and older men and women. It begins by discussing a final outcome: death. Though its timing differs for men and women, are the medical reasons for death usually the same? Then it concentrates on data about health in the many years before death, especially chronic conditions and associated disability for middle-aged and older adults. What is it like to be an older woman or man, with respect to daily symptoms, long-term experience of fatal and nonfatal chronic conditions, and limitations in physical and social activities? Are there special health problems for women or men those ages, or is similarity in their health problems the usual situation? What are the most central and pervasive differences in illness/disability between men and women? It concludes with comments about the dynamics of health, for individuals over their lifetimes and for populations as a whole, and how age and sex impel both kinds of dynamics.

Throughout the chapter, the terms age and sex are often used in a demographic way, simply to designate groups being compared. What actually causes the observed differences involves both social and biological features, thus gender and aging as well as sex and age. As readers consider *why* the differences exist, answers will spring from both social and biological domains.

Near the end of each section, references for further reading are noted. To keep the lists short, they are mainly review articles (with plenty of detailed references therein), data sources with discussions, and selected research articles.

MORTALITY RATES AND TRENDS

Mortality Rates

The 1950s and 1960s were a period of relative stability in mortality rates in the United States, compared to protracted declines during the earlier decades of the century. Demographers and health planners felt that a stable "low" had been reached and further declines would not happen, since major medical or life-style changes were not expected to occur. To their surprise, mortality rates began to fall notably in the late 1960s, and they have continued downward since then. The reasons are not fully understood, but experts attribute the declines to improved medical care and drugs for circulatory diseases, wider access to medical services, and adoption of better life-styles (especially, less smoking and alcohol consumption, and improved diet and physical fitness).[1]

Older men and women (ages 65+) have experienced the largest declines, in absolute terms, with middle-aged people (ages 45-64) next. Table 1 shows the gains made at these ages across three decades: 1955-65, 1965-75, 1975-85. Note first how small the mortality improvements are in the 1955-65 decade compared to the subsequent two. It is worthwhile to look closely at the numbers for the recent decades. For example, for males (All Ages, Adjusted), 128 more persons per 100,000 stayed alive in 1985 than in 1975. That is a modest gain. But for males ages 65-69, 574 per 100,000 did not die in 1985, compared to their age peers in 1975. The "savings" are even larger for ages 70-74 and 75-79. Older women also show pronounced gains for the 1965-75 and 1975-85 intervals, larger than for All Ages or middle ones. For example, for females ages 70-74, the savings for 1965-75 and 1975-85 were 457 and 346 persons per 100,000, compared to 97 and 60 for All Ages, Adjusted.

Percentage declines are also presented in Table 2.1. They show that the relative (percentage) gains were roughly similar for middle-aged and older women, and slightly larger for middle-aged than older men. This happens because smaller absolute declines at middle ages are placed over a smaller rate (or stated differently, older people have larger declines over larger rates); the result can be rather similar percentage improvements. Relative gains are important in public health perspectives, since they help one judge progress in hard-won (low rates) territory vs. more easily won (high rates) territory. Our interest will tend to stay with absolute changes, since they offer a more direct view of how many people in the various age-sex groups stay in the living population as mortality improves.

Men's absolute gains have exceeded women's, except at advanced ages (75+). Starting at higher mortality levels, they have made more visible advances. This is especially true for white males (not shown in Table 2.1). Among all other races, women's gains have often surpassed men's, a signal of recalcitrant high risks among black and other non-white men.

TABLE 2.1 Mortality Rates and Changes in Rates, for U.S. Males and Females Ages 45+, 1955-1985

	Mortality Rates (Deaths per 100,000 Pop.)				Absolute Change (t_1-t_0)			Percentage Change ([t_1-t_0]/t_0 x 100)		
	1955	1965	1975	1985	1955 -65	1965 -75	1975 -85	1955 -65	1965 -75	1975 -85
Male										
45-49	756	743	667	514	- 13	- 76	-153	-1.7%	-10.2	-22.9
50-54	1226	1216	1044	836	- 10	-172	-208	-0.8	-14.1	-19.9
55-59	1842	1888	1615	1342	+ 46	-273	-273	+2.5	-14.5	-16.9
60-64	2736	2804	2523	2062	+ 68	-281	-461	+2.5	-10.0	-18.3
65-69	4015	4285	3636	3062	+270	-649	-574	+6.7	-15.1	-15.8
70-74	5747	6004	5556	4748	+257	-448	-808	+4.5	-7.5	-14.5
75-79	8545	8446	8254	7143	- 99	-192	-1111	-1.2	-2.3	-13.5
80-84	13035	12418	11593	11024	-607	-825	-569	-4.7	-6.6	-4.9
85+	19588	21279	17573	18325	+1691	-3706	+752	+8.6	-17.4	+4.3
All Ages	1077	1088	1013	945	- 11	- 75	- 68	-1.0	-6.9	-6.7
(Adjusted)[a]	934	944	845	717	+ 10	- 99	-128	+1.1	-10.5	-15.2

26

Female

45-49	433	423	366	286	-10	-57	-80	-2.3%	-13.5	-21.9
50-54	672	628	544	464	-44	-84	-80	-6.5	-13.4	-14.7
55-59	983	917	821	721	-66	-96	-100	-6.7	-10.5	-12.2
60-64	1492	1380	1227	1120	-112	-153	-107	-7.5	-11.1	-8.7
65-69	2390	2232	1731	1671	-158	-501	-60	-6.6	-22.4	-3.5
70-74	3770	3402	2945	2599	-368	-457	-346	-9.8	-13.4	-11.7
75-79	6378	5582	4879	4094	-796	-703	-785	-12.5	-12.6	-16.1
80-84	10292	9475	7687	6958	-817	-1788	-729	-7.9	-18.9	-9.5
85+	18555	19526	14031	14343	+971	-5495	+312	+5.2	-28.1	+2.2
All Ages	788	803	770	807	+15	-33	+37	+1.9	-4.1	+4.8
(Adjusted)	607	566	469	409	-41	-97	-60	-6.8	-17.1	-12.8

SOURCE: For 1955: Unpublished rates on file at the National Center for Health Statistics. Age-adjusted rate for 1955 from Klebba, Maurer, and Glass (1973). For 1965: *Vital Statistics of the United States*, Vol. II, Part A. For 1975: *Monthly Vital Statistics Report*, 25 (11, Supplement). For 1985: *Monthly Vital Statistics Report*, 36 (5, Supplement).
Rates and changes for white and all other races are available from the author.

a. Adjusted to the age distribution of the total U.S. population enumerated in 1940.

All middle-aged and older groups have had mortality improvements in the past two decades, except the very oldest group (85+: declines for 1965-75 but then increases for 1975-85). The recent rises may be due to either an increase in average age of the group (this automatically elevates mortality rates even though single-age rates stay constant) or an increasing average frailty among them (frail people of all ages are retained in the population more than in prior decades, but they die with rapidity once they reach very advanced ages).[2]

Life Expectancy

Life expectancy is a useful summary of mortality rates in a given year. Table 2.2 shows life expectancies at middle and older age points, as well as at birth, in recent decades. These state the average number of years of life remaining for people at age x, as of the calendar year shown. Women have higher life expectancy at all ages, though their margin becomes quite small—just a year or so—at the very oldest ages.

The absolute gains in life expectancy are especially remarkable for middle-aged people: men and women at age 45 in 1985 can each expect 2.9 more years of life than their age peers in 1965. No matter which decade we look at, improvements are smaller as age advances, but they still exist (except for 85+ recently). Which sex has made the greatest gains? Though women had larger improvements from 1965-75, the more recent decade shows *men* making similar or larger gains. That is a new phenomenon; we have witnessed periods of equal and large gains for *women* during this century, up to that.

Relative gains have been distinctly larger for middle-aged and older persons than for newborns. For example, men at age 65 gained 6.6 percent, compared to just 3.6 percent at birth; the figures for women are 3.3 percent and 2.2 percent.

A convincing demonstration of how sizable the improvements for adults are, and how gains are concentrated in older ages, comes from bounded life expectancies (also called temporary life expectancy). These state how many years in a specific age interval someone alive at its start can expect to live (Table 2.3). (By contrast, all the numbers in Table 2.2 are open-ended, with no upper age bound.) For the interval from birth to age 20, males gained .38 a year from 1960-80, and females .28, due largely to declines in infant mortality. Improvements for the 45-65 age interval were similar to this. But for the 65-85 age interval, males gained .76 a year and females 1.24. Projections for

TABLE 2.2 Expectation of Life at Birth, Middle, and Older Ages, for U.S. Males and Females, 1955-1985

	Life Expectancy (Average No. of Years of Life Remaining at Age x)[a]				*Absolute Change* $(t_1\text{-}t_0)$			*Percentage Change* $([t_1\text{-}t_0]/t_0 \times 100)$		
	1955	*1965*	*1975*	*1985*	*1955 -65*	*1965 -75*	*1975 -85*	*1955 -65*	*1965 -75*	*1975 -85*
Male										
e_0	66.7	66.8	68.7	71.2	+ 0.1	+1.9	+ 2.5	+0.1%	+2.8	+3.6
e_{45}	27.2	27.0	28.3	29.9	− 0.2	+ 1.3	+ 1.6	−0.7	+4.8	+5.7
e_{55}	19.5	19.2	20.3	21.6	− 0.3	+ 1.1	+ 1.3	−1.6	+5.7	+6.4
e_{65}	13.1	12.9	13.7	14.6	− 0.2	+ 0.8	+ 0.9	−1.5	+6.2	+6.6
e_{70}	10.5	10.4	10.9	11.5	− 0.1	+ 0.5	+ 0.6	−1.0	+4.8	+5.5
e_{75}	8.1	8.1	8.6	9.0	+ 0.0	+ 0.5	+ 0.4	+0.0	+6.2	+4.7
e_{80}	6.2	6.2	6.8	6.8	+ 0.0	+ 0.6	+ 0.0	+0.0	+9.7	+0.0
e_{85}	4.9	4.5	5.4	5.1	− 0.4	+ 0.9	− 0.3	−8.2	+20.0	−5.6
Female										
e_0	72.8	73.7	76.5	78.2	+ 0.9	+ 2.8	+ 1.7	+1.2	+3.8	+2.2
e_{45}	31.8	32.5	34.5	35.4	+ 0.7	+ 2.0	+ 0.9	+2.2	+6.2	+2.6
e_{55}	23.3	24.0	25.8	26.5	+ 0.7	+ 1.8	+ 0.7	+3.0	+7.5	+2.7
e_{65}	15.6	16.2	18.0	18.6	+ 0.6	+ 1.8	+ 0.6	+3.8	+11.1	+3.3
e_{70}	12.3	12.8	14.4	14.9	+ 0.5	+ 1.6	+ 0.5	+4.1	+12.5	+3.5
e_{75}	9.4	9.7	11.3	11.7	+ 0.3	+ 1.6	+ 0.4	+3.2	+16.5	+3.5
e_{80}	7.0	7.0	8.7	8.8	+ 0.0	+ 1.7	+ 0.1	+0.0	+24.3	+1.1
e_{85}	5.1	4.8	6.7	6.4	− 0.3	+ 1.9	− 0.3	−5.9	+39.6	−4.5

SOURCE: For 1955: Unpublished life tables on file at the National Center for Health Statistics. For 1965, 1975, 1985: *Vital Statistics of the United States*, (Year), Vol. I.
Data for white and all other races are available from the author.
a. From abridged life tables. Average years remaining at start of age interval (0-1 for e_0, x to x+5 for the other e_x).

1980-2000 show notably larger gains for middle-aged and older people than for children.

Any future gains in mortality virtually must occur at older ages; there is almost no room left for improvement elsewhere. For example, a person at age 20 who asks how many years of the next 25 he or she can expect to live gets a remarkable answer: 24.5 years for men, 24.8 for women (Table 2.3, projected 1990). By contrast, someone at age 65 asking about the next 20 years learns that the expectation is currently 13.4 for men and 16.1 for women.

TABLE 2.3 Bounded Life Expectancies for U.S. Males and Females, 1960-2000

	Bounded Life Expectancy (Average No. of Years of Life in Age Interval)				Absolute Change $(t_1 - t_0)$	
	1960	1980	1990[a]	2000[a]	1960 -80	1980 -2000
Male						
Birth to age 20	19.24	19.62	19.71	19.73	0.38	0.11
20-45	24.37	24.35	24.46	24.50	−0.02	0.15
45-65	17.77	18.23	18.55	18.69	0.46	0.46
65-85	12.00	12.76	13.42	13.76	0.76	1.00
Female						
Birth to age 20	19.43	19.71	19.78	19.80	0.28	0.09
20-45	24.67	24.76	24.81	24.82	0.09	0.06
45-65	18.78	19.04	19.19	19.26	0.26	0.22
65-85	14.26	15.50	16.11	16.40	1.24	0.90

SOURCE: From Olshansky and Ault (1986: Table 2). Calculated by them from data in J.F. Faber, *Life Tables for the United States: 1900-2050*, Actuarial Study No. 87, (SSA Publ. No. 11-11534), Social Security Administration, Washington, D.C. (now superseded by later issue).

a. Projected for 1990 and 2000.

The mortality rates and life expectancies all indicate that people are surviving longer. Most gain a few additional years of life, and this pushes up the mean age of death for decedents a little (Olshansky & Ault, 1986, Figure 3). Stated another way, survival curves shift to the right. (Survival curves show proportions of a starting population still alive, at every age from zero on up.) But beyond this, the ability of some persons to endure to very advanced ages has also increased. In 1950, one percent of males could expect to be still alive at age 95.1; for women, the age was 97.5 (Faber & Wade, 1983, Table 6). In 1980, the figures had risen to 97.4 for males and 101.6 for females. Thus, the "tail" of survival curves is stretching out to the right for both sexes, tapering off more slowly. There is no sign yet that the recent mortality improvements are bumping up against some intrinsic limits to human life span.[3]

Mortality Trends

Age causes the largest differentials in mortality rates, but sex comes next, ahead of any other sociodemographic characteristics. Throughout this century, females have had lower overall mortality rates (and higher life expectancy) than males. The gap widened especially after World War II, as men's improvements stagnated while women's slowly continued (Figure 2.1). In the 1970s, the sex ratio of (age-adjusted) rates stood at 1.75-1.80; that is, men's rates were about 75-80 percent higher than women's. There were signs in the 1970s that the pace of increase in women's advantage was slowing, and that the gap might stabilize or even narrow (Verbrugge, 1980). The 1980s are confirming this fundamentally new situation. The sex difference (F-M) in life expectancy has decreased slightly, and so has the sex ratio (M/F) of mortality rates (Table 2.4). (The peak sex ratio, 1.80, was recorded in 1975, 1977, 1978, and 1979.) This is due both to women's failure to sustain their mortality gains and to especially strong recent advances by men (see Table 2.1). It is widely held that women are now suffering the consequences of post-World War II increases in smoking behavior. Projections for the future are that the sex mortality ratio will stabilize, or still widen a little but never at the pace experienced in mid-century (Faber & Wade, 1983; Olshansky & Ault, 1986).

Leading Causes of Death

Sex ratios for leading causes of death are shown in Table 2.5. Men have higher mortality from all of the causes except diabetes mellitus. Their excess is especially great for cardiovascular (All Ages: 1.95) and respiratory diseases (COPD, 2.23), chronic liver disease (2.23), and external causes (2.78 for accidents, 3.84 for suicide, and 3.28 for homicide). (Diabetes is a genuine anomaly, the only disease of public health importance with virtually no sex difference in mortality rates.) Across middle and older ages, the overall (All Causes) sex difference narrows.[4] This occurs for most specific titles too: diseases of heart, cerebrovascular diseases, accidents, pneumonia/influenza, diabetes slightly, atherosclerosis, homicide, chronic liver disease. The narrowing is due to faster-paced mortality increases with age among women

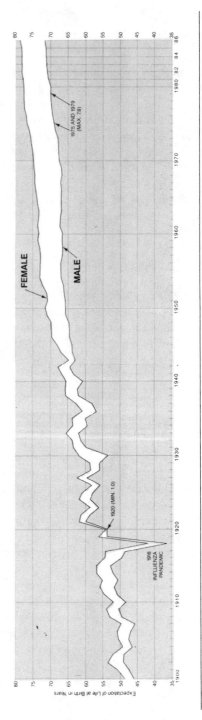

Figure 2.1. Trends in Expectation of Life at Birth for Males and Females, U. S., 1900-1986.

SOURCE: *Statistical Bulletin*, Vol. 68. No. 3 (July.-Sept. 1987), Metropolitan Life Insurance Co.

TABLE 2.4 Sex Differentials in Mortality, United States, 1965-1985

	Age-Adjusted Mortality Rates (per 100,000 pop.)[a]				
	1965	*1970*	*1975*	*1980*	*1985*
Male	944	932	845	777	717
Female	566	532	469	433	409
Ratio (M/F)	1.67	1.75	1.80	1.79	1.75
	Expectation of Life at Birth				
	1965	*1970*	*1975*	*1980*	*1985*
Male	66.8	67.1	68.7	70.0	71.2
Female	73.7	74.8	76.5	77.5	78.2
Difference (F–M)	6.9	7.7	7.8	7.5	7.0

SOURCE: For age-adjusted mortality 1965, 1975, 1985: See Sources in Table 2.1; for 1970, 1980: *Vital Statistics of the United States*, Vol. II, Part A. For expectation of life, all years shown: *Vital Statistics of the United States*, (Year), Vol. I.

a. Adjusted to the age distribution of the total U.S. population enumerated in 1940.

(for the first six titles) or slow declines for them (for homicide) (liver disease has a nonlinear pattern). A few titles do show widening sex differences with age (malignant neoplasms, COPD, suicide, nephritis/nephrosis), due uniformly to faster increases among men with age.

Men and women die from fundamentally the same causes, even though their rates differ. In other words, the pace of death differs much more than the reasons. Table 2.6 shows the leading causes of death for men and women in various age groups. In a given age span, the lists for men and women are very similar, especially after age 55.[5] The main differences (by ranks) are the larger importance of malignant neoplasms for middle-aged women than same-age men; the lesser importance for women of heart diseases (in middle ages only), suicide, and homicide; and the slightly greater importance of diabetes for women. Note that across ages for both sexes, the importance (ranks) of septicemia, pneumonia/influenza, and atherosclerosis rise, while ranks for chronic liver disease and external causes fall. The three ascending titles are conditions that reflect overall physical frailty—the body's vulnerability to severe acute conditions and general wearing out of the cardiovascular system. It makes good sense to see these rise with age.

TABLE 2.5 Sex Ratios of Mortality Rates for Leading Causes of Death, United States, 1985

Cause of Death	Rank of Mortality Rate[a,b]			Sex Ratio (M/F)					
	All Ages	45-64	65+	All Ages[c]	45-54	55-64	65-74	75-84	85+
All causes	—	—	—	1.75	1.80	1.84	1.81	1.63	1.28
Diseases of heart	1	2	1	1.95	3.21	2.60	2.02	1.56	1.17
Malignant neoplasms	2	1	2	1.48	1.06	1.40	1.68	1.94	1.91
Cerebrovascular diseases (CVD)	3	3	3	1.17	1.20	1.34	1.31	1.16	0.90
Accidents and adverse effects	4	4	7	2.78	2.94	2.62	1.84	1.80	1.69
COPD and allied conditions[d]	5	5	4	2.23	1.23	1.66	2.25	3.07	3.63
Pneumonia and influenza	6	9	5	1.80	1.90	2.10	2.10	1.84	1.49
Diabetes mellitus	7	7	6	1.05	1.24	1.02	1.01	1.01	0.94
Suicide	8	8	13	3.84	2.83	3.48	4.83	7.81	12.04
Chronic liver disease & cirrhosis	9	6	11	2.23	2.32	2.34	2.04	1.82	1.76
Atherosclerosis	10	16	8	1.31	2.40	2.28	1.78	1.24	0.97
Nephritis, nephrotic syndrome, and nephrosis	11	11	9	1.52	1.25	1.31	1.48	1.62	1.81
Homicide & legal interventions	12	10	21	3.28	3.56	3.37	2.46	1.71	1.29
Septicemia	14	12	10	1.40	1.46	1.54	1.62	1.35	1.19

SOURCE: Ranks are determined from *Monthly Vital Statistics Report*, 36 (5, Supplement), Tables 7 and 8. Ratios are calculated from unpublished mortality rates for 1985 provided by the National Center for Health Statistics (now published in *Vital Statistics of the United States*).

a. The top-ten titles for All Ages (both sexes) are shown. They cover most leading causes for the age groups 45-64 and 65+ as well. Several titles (nephritis, homicide, septicemia), which rank in the top ten for an age group, but not All Ages, are also included.
b. Other diseases of arteries/arterioles/capillaries (ICD 441–448) cause a sizable number of deaths, but the title is viewed as a residual category and usually not ranked. If ranked, it would be the eleventh leading cause for All Ages, tenth for 45-64, and ninth for 65+.
c. Based on age-adjusted rates.
d. Chronic obstructive pulmonary diseases; includes chronic bronchitis, emphysema, asthma, other.

The descending titles are conditions closely related to life-style behaviors, which have "room" in middle ages to levy a strong toll before chronic diseases assert themselves forcefully at later ages.

The principal cause of higher mortality for middle-aged men is heart disease, which accounts for over 50 percent of the male excess (Table 2.7). In older ages, higher rates of malignant neoplasms and heart diseases are the chief reasons for men's higher mortality. Overall, as age increases, the contributions of malignant neoplasms, pneumonia/influenza, and COPD to the sex difference rise, while those of heart diseases and external causes (accidents, suicide, homicide) fall. Thus, in late life (85+), just four problems cause the great majority (83%) of males' excess mortality: malignant neoplasms, heart diseases, pnuemonia/influenza, and COPD. Readers are encouraged to look at the numbers in Table 2.7 carefully to get a good view of the causes of men's "extra" mortality at various ages.

REFERENCES: For further reading on sex mortality differentials and trends, see Crimmins, 1981, 1984; Fingerhut, 1982; Klebba, Maurer, & Glass, 1973; McMillen & Rosenberg, 1983; Metropolitan Life Insurance Co., 1987, 1988; Nathanson, 1984; Olshansky & Ault, 1986; Rosenwaike, 1985a; Rosenwaike, Yaffe, & Sagi, 1980; Verbrugge, 1976a, 1980; Verbrugge & Wingard, 1987; Waldron, 1976.

Explanations for Sex Mortality Differences

Why do women live longer than men? Underlying social and biological reasons for women's mortality advantage have been discussed extensively (Hazzard, 1984; Holden, 1987; Lopez & Ruzicka, 1983; Nathanson, 1984; Verbrugge, 1976a; Verbrugge & Wingard, 1987; Waldron, 1982, 1983a, 1986a; Wingard, 1984). Precise empirical reasons for it are investigated in several studies (Preston, 1976; Retherford, 1975; Waldron, 1986b; Wingard, 1982; Wingard, Suarez, & Barrett-Connor, 1983).

Here, we shall state a broad conclusion of those efforts. Men's life-styles (smoking, alcohol consumption, and driving behavior) and their tendency to express distress and anger in violent behaviors toward self and others are prominent reasons for their excess mortality—but not sufficient reasons. There is both theoretical and empirical evidence for greater intrinsic (genetic or hormonal) robustness among females. Thus, even if males and females had, on average, similar lifetime risk exposures and physical responsiveness to those risks, there would still

TABLE 2.6 Leading Causes of Death for U.S. Men and Women, in Middle and Older Ages, 1985

(Deaths per 100,000 Population)

Rank[a]	Men 45-54	Women 45-54
1	Diseases of heart, 237	Malignant neoplasms, 164
2	Malignant neoplasms, 174	Diseases of heart, 74
3	Accidents (and adverse effects), 47	Cerebrovascular diseases, 19
4	Chronic liver disease/cirrhosis, 31	Accidents, 16
5	Suicide, 24	Chronic liver disease/cirrhosis, 13
6	Cerebrovascular diseases, 23	COPD, 9
7	Homicide (and legal interv.), 13	Suicide, 8
8	COPD, 11	Diabetes mellitus, 8
9	Diabetes mellitus, 10	Pneumonia/influenza, 5
10	Pneumonia/influenza, 10	Homicide, 4
	Men 55-64	*Women 55-64*
1	Diseases of heart, 652	Malignant neoplasms, 379
2	Malignant neoplasms, 531	Diseases of heart, 250
3	Cerebrovascular diseases, 63	Cerebrovascular diseases, 47
4	COPD, 60	COPD, 36
5	Accidents, 54	Diabetes mellitus, 26
6	Chronic liver disease/cirrhosis, 48	Accidents, 21
7	Suicide, 27	Chronic liver disease/cirrhosis, 21
8	Diabetes mellitus, 26	Pneumonia/influenza, 12
9	Pneumonia/influenza, 26	Nephritis/nephrosis, 8
10	Nephritis/nephrosis, 11	Suicide, 8
	Men 65-74	*Women 65-74*
1	Diseases of heart, 1508	Diseases of heart, 745
2	Malignant neoplasms, 1086	Malignant neoplasms, 645
3	COPD, 215	Cerebrovascular diseases, 150
4	Cerebrovascular diseases, 198	COPD, 95
5	Pneumonia/influenza, 82	Diabetes mellitus, 59
6	Accidents, 68	Pneumonia/influenza, 39
7	Diabetes mellitus, 60	Accidents, 37
8	Chronic liver disease/cirrhosis, 52	Chronic liver disease/cirrhosis, 26
9	Nephritis/nephrosis, 34	Nephritis/nephrosis, 23
10	Suicide, 33	Septicemia, 17

(continued)

TABLE 2.6 Continued

	(Deaths per 100,000 Population)	
Rank[a]	Men 75-84	Women 75-84
1	Diseases of heart, 3498	Diseases of heart, 2245
2	Malignant neoplasms, 1840	Malignant neoplasms, 948
3	Cerebrovascular diseases, 661	Cerebrovascular diseases, 573
4	COPD, 505	Pneumonia/influenza, 184
5	Pneumonia/influenza, 338	COPD, 164
6	Accidents, 149	Diabetes mellitus, 128
7	Diabetes mellitus, 129	Accidents, 83
8	Nephritis/nephrosis, 103	Atherosclerosis, 76
9	Atherosclerosis, 94	Nephritis/nephrosis, 64
10	Septicemia, 74	Septicemia, 54
	Men 85+	*Women 85+*
1	Diseases of heart, 8124	Diseases of heart, 6936
2	Malignant neoplasms, 2414	Cerebrovascular diseases, 1891
3	Cerebrovascular diseases, 1703	Malignant neoplasms, 1263
4	Pneumonia/influenza, 1339	Pneumonia/influenza, 897
5	COPD, 746	Atherosclerosis, 469
6	Atherosclerosis, 457	Diabetes mellitus, 219
7	Accidents, 359	Accidents, 213
8	Nephritis/nephrosis, 314	COPD, 206
9	Diabetes mellitus, 206	Nephritis/nephrosis, 174
10	Septicemia, 181	Septicemia, 151

SOURCE: Derived from unpublished mortality rates for 1985 provided by the National Center for Health Statistics (now published in *Vital Statistics of the United States*).

a. Ranks are based on 72 disease and injury titles, which encompass the International Classification of Diseases. Rates are rounded to integers for presentation here.

be a mortality gap. Based on information about causes of death that underly the sex differential and about risks that prompt those conditions, we judge social causes to be preeminent (90% or more of the gap), and biological ones quite minor, but also in women's favor.[6]

PHYSICAL HEALTH

Chronic illness is not a universal feature of late life, but it is certainly a common one. Prevalence rates of most fatal chronic conditions and

TABLE 2.7 Components of the Sex Mortality Difference, United States, 1985

	Ages 45-54		55-64		65-74		75-84		85+	
Cause of Death	*M-F*	*% of diff.*	*M-F*	*% of Diff.*	*M-F*	*% of Diff.*	*M-F*	*% of Diff.*	*M-F*	*% of Diff.*
All causes	296.5	—	773.6	—	1693.0	—	3284.3	—	3981.9	—
Septicemia	—	—	—	—	10.4	0.6	19.1	0.6	29.4	0.7
Malignant neoplasms	10.5	3.5	152.0	19.6	441.0	26.0	891.9	27.2	1150.8	28.9
Diabetes	1.9	0.6	0.6	0.1	0.8	0.0	1.1	0.0	-12.9	-0.3
Diseases of heart	163.1	55.0	401.6	51.9	763.1	45.1	1252.8	28.1	1188.0	29.8
Cerebrovascular dis.	3.8	1.3	16.0	2.1	47.3	2.8	88.7	2.7	-188.0	-4.7
Atherosclerosis	—	—	—	—	—	—	17.9	0.5	-12.7	-0.3
Pneumonia/influenza	4.5	1.5	13.4	1.7	43.0	2.5	154.6	4.7	441.9	11.1
COPD	2.1	0.7	23.8	3.1	119.6	7.1	340.9	10.4	540.7	13.6
Chron. liver dis. /cirrhosis	17.7	6.0	27.8	3.6	26.7	1.6	—	—	—	—
Nephritis/Nephrosis	—	—	2.6	0.3	10.9	0.6	39.2	1.2	140.5	3.5
Accidents[b]	31.3	10.6	33.7	4.4	31.1	1.8	66.4	2.0	146.1	3.7
Suicide[b]	15.2	5.1	19.1	2.5	26.4	1.6	—	—	—	—
Homicide[b]	9.2	3.1	—	—	—	—	—	—	—	—
(Subtotal for leading causes)	259.3	87.4%	690.6	89.3%	1520.3	89.7%	2872.6	87.4%	3423.8	86.0%
All other causes	37.2		83.0		172.7		411.7		558.1	

(Computed for the ten leading titles in each age group)[a]

SOURCE: Calculated from unpublished mortality rates for 1985 provided by the National Center for Health Statistics (now published in *Vital Statistics of the United States*).

— Not in the top ten causes for the age group.

a. Leading titles for each age group were determined from *Monthly Vital Statistics Report*, 36 (5, Supplement), Table 8. Titles on the left are listed in the order of the International Classification of Diseases. Finding the components is a simple algebra exercise, first computing sex differences (M-F) for selected causes and then percentaging them over the total sex difference.

b. The share of the excess due to external causes (accidents, suicide, homicide) for the five age groups is: 18.8%, 7.7, 3.6, 3.5, 5.0.

nonfatal ones (these include diseases and also structural/sensory impairments) rise steeply from middle age onward.

Leading Chronic Conditions

The leading chronic conditions at ages 45-64 are a mixture of nonfatal problems, precursors to fatal ones (such as high blood pressure), and just a few fatal conditions (such as ischemic heart disease for men and diabetes for both sexes) (Table 2.8). With increasing age, fatal circulatory conditions become more prominent. Still, the lists remain dominated by nonfatal impairments and diseases, especially women's. With age, skeletal impairments diminish in importance while sensory ones become more so.[7]

For women, arthritis and high blood pressure stand out as the foremost problems in middle and older ages. Rates for all the other leading conditions are much lower. But even the top two have a distinct hierarchy for women: arthritis rates surpass by a good distance those for hypertension.[8] Arthritis is less dominant in men's lives. It ranks as the second problem for middle-aged and elderly (ages 75+) men, and barely first at ages 65-74. One condition is clearly more prominent in men's than in women's lives: ischemic heart disease. Its rank, and rate, are higher at all ages among men.

The differential importance of arthritis and heart disease constitutes the key sex difference in leading conditions (ranks). Looking more generally at the lists, the presence of fatal problems there increases much more sharply for men with age than for women. So, men's and women's lists differ most at ages 75+.

Combing for sex differences can make us ignore the most basic conclusion, that the lists of leading conditions (the titles that appear there) are really very similar for the sexes. What bothers one sex bothers the other as well, even though the specific ranks may differ. This is the theme; the differences noted above are the variation on that theme.[9]

Focusing on ranks masks an important and persistent facet of women's lives, their more frequent experience of illness, symptoms, and ensuing health care. For the large majority of *nonfatal* chronic diseases, women's prevalence rates exceed men's (Table 2.9).[10] Men have higher rates for relatively few nonfatal conditions, mostly sensory and orthopedic impairments. The situation completely reverses for *fatal* conditions (Table 2.10). Here, men consistently have excess rates

TABLE 2.8 Leading Chronic Conditions, for Age-Sex Groups, 1983-1985, United States

(Conditions per 1,000 persons. Average annual rate.)[a,b]

MEN, 45-64			WOMEN, 45-64	
1	High blood pressure, 254	'F'	Arthritis, 339	N
2	Arthritis, 214	N	High blood pressure, 274	'F'
3	Hearing impairment, 196	I	Chronic sinusitis, 198	N
4	Chronic sinusitis, 163	N	Hearing impairment, 106	I
5	Ischemic heart disease, 87	F	Hay fever without asthma, 98	N
6	Def./orth, impairment[c]-back, 87	I	Def./orth. impairment-back, 95	I
7	Hay fever without asthma, 79	N	Varicose veins, 88	N
8	Hemorrhoids 76	N	Hemorrhoids, 72	N
9	Def./orth. imp.-lower extrem., 72	I	Chronic bronchitis, 65	'F'
10	Visual impairment, 62	I	Migraine headache, 59	N
11	Diabetes, 52	F	Diabetes, 57	F
12	Tinnitus, 51	N	Bursitis, 54	N
13	Hernia of abdominal cavity, 45	N	Def./orth. imp.-lower extrem., 53	I
14	Bursitis, 41	N	Heart rhythm disorders, 48	N
15	Intervertebral disc disorders, 41	I	Corns and calluses, 47	N

MEN, 65-74			WOMEN, 65-74	
1	Arthritis, 371	N	Arthritis, 528	N
2	High blood pressure, 349	'F'	High blood pressure, 454	'F'
3	Hearing impairment, 318	I	Hearing impairment, 216	I
4	Ischemic heart disease, 190	F	Chronic sinusitis, 182	N
5	Chronic sinusitis, 147	N	Cataracts, 125	N
6	Tinnitus, 90	N	Ischemic heart disease, 114	F
7	Diabetes, 90	F	Diabetes, 104	F
8	Visual impairment, 83	I	Varicose veins, 100	N
9	Other selected heart diseases, 79	F	Def./orth. impairment-back, 100	I
10	Atherosclerosis, 77	F	Tinnitus, 91	N
11	Def./orth. impairment-back, 77	I	Hemorrhoids, 82	N
12	Hemorrhoids, 75	N	Heart rhythm disorders, 81	N
13	Emphysema, 73	F	Chronic bronchitis, 80	'F'
14	Hernia of abdominal cavity, 71	N	Def./orth. imp.-lower extrem., 80	I
15	Def./orth. imp.-lower extrem., 64	I	Hernia of abdominal cavity, 75	N

TABLE 2.8 Continued

(Conditions per 1,000 persons. Average annual rate.)[a,b]

	MEN, 75+		WOMEN, 75+	
1	Hearing impairment, 447	I	Arthritis, 566	N
2	Arthritis, 405	N	High blood pressure, 459	'F'
3	High blood pressure, 286	. 'F'	Hearing impairment, 343	I
4	Cataracts, 178	N	Cataracts, 278	N
5	Ischemic heart disease, 158	F	Chronic sinusitis, 153	N
6	Visual impairment, 144	I	Visual impairment, 132	I
7	Chronic sinusitis, 128	N	Ischemic heart disease, 130	F
8	Atherosclerosis, 111	F	Frequent constipation, 119	N
9	Other selected heart diseases, 104	F	Atherosclerosis, 110	F
10	Cerebrovascular disease, 98	F	Varicose veins, 109	N
11	Diabetes, 93	F	Heart rhythm disorders, 108	N
12	Tinnitus, 79	N	Other selected heart diseases, 107	F
13	Emphysema, 79	F	Def./orth. imp.-back, 101	I
14	Frequent constipation, 76	N	Diabetes, 91	F
15	Diseases of prostate[d], 76	F	Def./orth. imp.-lower extrem., 89	I

SOURCE: Calculated from unpublished data for the National Health Interview Survey, 1983-85, provided by the National Center for Health Statistics.

a. The titles originate in six lists of specific conditions, queried to sampled households (one list per household). The lists cover high prevalence conditions and other selected conditions of public health importance, but exclude mental disorders. Rates for 95 titles, encompassing all chronic conditions (except mental) in the International Classification of Diseases, were computed and evaluated for ranks. They are rounded to integers for presentation. All rates shown here have low sampling error (relative standard error 30% or less).

b. On the right of each column, conditions are noted with I for impairment, N for nonfatal disease, and F for fatal disease. ('F' is for hypertension and chronic bronchitis; see footnotes in Table 2.10.) Conditions potentially fatal but rarely so now score N.

c. Deformity or orthopedic impairment.

d. Includes cancer.

(there are occasional age groups with a small female excess). Just three titles have clearly higher female rates, and readers should see the footnotes in Table 2.10 for comments about them. In sum, Tables 2.9 and 2.10 offer striking evidence of women's greater burden from non-fatal diseases and men's from fatal diseases and many impairments. Men's lives are shortened by their higher rates of fatal illnesses. Women's lives are filled with bothersome symptoms of nonfatal ones, due possibly to higher chances of developing the conditions at a given age (incidence) and certainly to more total years enduring their progression (duration).

TABLE 2.9 Sex Ratios (F/M) for Selected Nonfatal Chronic Conditions, 1983-1985, United States

	Age: 45-64	65-74	75+
Arthritis	1.59	1.43	1.40
Sciatica	1.85	1.25	1.30*
Bunion	4.36	3.48*	3.34*
Bursitis	1.31	1.29	1.37
Dermatitis	1.59	1.62	1.76
Trouble with corns and calluses	1.82	1.65	2.63
Def./orth. impairment-back	1.09	1.31	1.89
Cataracts	1.11	2.06	1.56
Diseases of retina	1.32	1.22*	1.32*
Gallstones	1.64	2.55*	1.43*
Gastritis and duodenitis	1.54	1.48	1.89*
Chronic enteritis and colitis	2.12	2.62*	2.58*
Spastic colon	4.05	6.24*	2.25*
Diverticula of intestines	2.52	2.30	2.27
Frequent constipation	3.53	2.83	1.56
Thyroid diseases	6.51	5.16*	3.43*
Anemias	4.78	1.75	2.88*
Migraine headache	2.75	2.97*	2.45*
Neuralgia and neuritis	1.79	1.99	1.15*
Bladder infection/disorders	4.82	2.37	2.06
Heart rhythm disorders	1.43	1.42	1.65
Varicose veins	3.33	2.50	2.23
Hay fever without asthma	1.23	1.23	1.11
Chronic sinusitis	1.23	1.24	1.19
BUT:			
Intervertebral disc disorders	0.86	0.72	0.86*
Visual impairments	0.51	0.77	0.91
Hearing impairments	0.54	0.68	0.77
Absence of upper/lower extrem.	0.21*	0.29	0.22*
Paralysis, complete or partial	0.75	0.71	1.03
Tinnitus	0.79	1.01	0.93
Hernia of abdominal cavity	0.82	1.06	0.98
Hemorrhoids	0.95	1.09	0.93

SOURCE: Calculated from unpublished data for the National Health Interview Survey, 1983-85, provided by the National Center for Health Statistics.
* High relative standard error (over 30%) for one or both rates.

TABLE 2.10 Sex Ratios (F/M) for Selected Fatal Chronic Conditions, 1983-1985, United States

	Age: 45-64	65-74	75+
Ischemic heart disease	0.49	0.60	0.82
Other selected heart diseases	0.97	0.86	1.03
Cerebrovascular disease	0.68	0.55	0.78
Atherosclerosis	0.46	0.77	0.99
Malignant neop. of lung/bronchus	0.71*	1.00*	0.36*
Asthma[c]	1.41	0.92	0.82
Emphysema	0.41	0.34	0.16
Ulcer of stomach/duodenum	0.97	0.69	1.44
Liver disease incl. cirrhosis	0.77	0.40*	0.47*
BUT:			
Diabetes[a]	1.11	1.16	0.98
High blood pressure[b]	1.08	1.30	1.61
Chronic bronchitis[c]	1.96	1.59	1.13

SOURCE: Calculated from unpublished data for the National Health Interview Survey, 1983-85, provided by the National Center for Health Statistics.
*High relative standard error (over 30%) for one or both rates.
a. Death rates from diabetes are also similar for men and women (see Table 2.5).
b. A risk factor for fatal circulatory diseases. Women's higher prevalence rates are thought to reflect earlier diagnosis and control, compared to men.
c. Fatal in severe forms; most cases are bothersome but have low fatality risk.

Daily Symptoms

Prevalence rates give a pale view of human suffering from chronic conditions. They simply indicate the presence of disease, not its severity or symptomatic nature. What symptoms pervade daily life and how frequent are they? Two community-based studies, in which respondents kept daily records of symptoms, concur that musculoskeletal symptoms dominate for both men and women (Table 2.11, top panel).[11] About half of them are attributed to disease (largely arthritis), and the other half to nondisease (overexertion, strain/sprain, etc.).[12] All other kinds of symptoms are much less frequent than musculoskeletal ones, and their rankings vary in the two studies. Both studies show the relatively small importance of cardiovascular symptoms in daily life, even though they are ultimately harbingers of death for many people.

TABLE 2.11 Daily Symptoms for Middle-Aged and Older Adults

(Based on prospective health diaries. Two community studies.)
Major Groups of Symptoms[a]

Detroit[b]	*(Average No. of Symptoms in 6-Week Period)*
Rank Men 45-64	Women 45-64

Rank	Men 45-64	Women 45-64
1	Musculoskeletal, 5.5	Musculoskeletal, 16.5
2	Respiratory, 4.8	Respiratory, 9.8
3	General[c] 2.2	Nervous system, 4.9
4	Nervous system, 2.2	General, 3.7
5	Digestive, 1.7	Digestive, 3.1
6	Skin, nails, and hair, 0.5	Psychological, 2.9
7	Psychological[d], 0.4	Eyes and ears, 1.7
8	Eyes and ears, 0.3	Genitourinary, 1.2
9	Cardiovascular,* Genitourinary,*	Skin, nails, and hair, 0.5
10	—	Cardiovascular, 0.2
	(N=59 diary-keepers)	(N=98)

	Men 65+	*Women 65+*
1	Musculoskeletal, 19.4	Musculoskeletal, 13.7
2	General 6.3	Respiratory, 7.7
3	Skin, nails, and hair, 5.5	General, 4.8
4	Respiratory, 5.0	Eyes and ears, 3.6
5	Eyes and ears, 3.6	Nervous system, 3.2
6	Digestive, 3.1	Psychological, 2.3
7	Nervous system, 1.6	Cardiovascular, 1.9
8	Cardiovascular, 0.8	Digestive, 1.8
9	Genitourinary, 0.7	Genitourinary, 1.5
10	Psychological, 0.7	Skin, nails, and hair, 0.2
	(N=27)	(N=35)

Southfield[e]	*(Average No. of Symptoms in 2-Week Period)*
Rank[f] Men 62+	Women 62+

Rank[f]	Men 62+	Women 62+
1	Musculoskeletal, 39.9	Musculoskeletal, 37.6
2	Eyes and ears, 15.0	Respiratory, 17.7
3	Respiratory, 11.6	Digestive, 9.5
4	Nervous system, 7.1	General, 8.6
5	Digestive, 6.3	Nervous system, 7.9
6	Psychological, 6.1	Eyes and ears, 7.7
7	Cardiovascular, 4.9	Psychological, 4.2
8	Skin, nails, and hair, 4.3	Cardiovascular, 2.6
9	General, 3.8	Skin, nails, and hair, 2.3
10	Genitourinary, 1.1	Genitourinary, 1.8
	(N=60 diary-keepers)	(N=82)

(continued)

TABLE 2.11 Continued

Specific Symptoms[g]

Detroit[h]		*(Percent of All Symptoms)*	
Rank	*Men 45-64*	*Women 45-64*	
1	Headache, 13.2%	Nerv	Headache, 9.7%	Nerv
2	Nasal congestion, 7.6	Resp	Back trouble, 6.7	Musc
3	Leg trouble, 7.1	Musc	Knee trouble, 5.5	Musc
4	Tiredness; Knee trouble, 7.0	Gen;Musc	Tension/nervousness, 5.4	Psych
5	Cough, 4.2	Resp	Joint pain, unspecified, 5.1	Musc
6	Neck trouble;	Musc	Sinus problems;	Resp;
	Back trouble, 4.0		Leg trouble, 4.6	Musc
7	Sore throat, 3.4	Resp	Tiredness, 4.1	Gen
8	Generalized pain;	Gen;Musc	Nasal congestion, 4.1	Resp
	Hand/finger trouble, 2.3			
	Tension/nervousness, 2.2	Psych	Neck trouble, 3.9	Musc
9	—		Cough, 3.2	Resp
10	(N=919 symptoms reported)		(N=3818)	

	Men 65+		*Women 65+*	
1	Leg trouble, 11.0%	Musc	Knee trouble, 8.8%	Musc
2	Skin irritation, 8.0	Skin	Leg trouble, 8.2	Musc
3	Hand/finger trouble, 6.9	Musc	Tiredness, 8.1	Gen
4	Generalized pain, 5.6	Gen	Back trouble, 7.4	Musc
5	Back trouble, 5.2	Musc	Tension/nervousness, 6.0	Psych
6	Foot/toe trouble, 5.1	Musc	Nasal congestion, 5.6	Resp
7	Shoulder trouble, 4.4	Musc	Circulation problems, 4.8	Circ
8	Knee trouble, 4.1	Musc	Headache, 4.5	Nerv
9	Chest area pain (excl. heart), 4.0	Gen	Shoulder trouble, 4.2	Musc
10	Hip trouble, 3.0	Musc	Eye problems (allergy, swelling), 3.6	Eye/ear
	(N=1218)		(N=1256)	

SOURCE: Health In Detroit Study, 1978; and Needs of the Elderly Study III, 1984.
* Less than 0.1

—No further major groups; or, all further specific symptoms have small n (less than 20 reports).
General Note: Titles are given the same rank if their sample n's are identical.

CAUTION: Comparisons of rates across the two studies is not recommended, since their strategies of eliciting symptoms differed (open-ended for Detroit, close-ended for Southfield).

a. Symptoms are coded according to the Reason for Visit Classification, developed for the National Ambulatory Medical Care Survey (Schneider et al., 1979).
b. The Health in Detroit Study had a probability sample of white adult (ages 18+) residents of the Detroit metropolitan area. They kept daily health records for 6 weeks in Fall 1978. Data are standardized to 6 weeks for each person to adjust for dropout.
c. General symptoms are whole-body problems such as tiredness, edema, generalized pain/ache all over, weakness, and general malaise.

(continued)

TABLE 2.11 Continued

Southfield[i]		*(Percent of All Symptoms)*	
Rank Men 62+		Women 62+	
1	Pain in joint/bones, 16.3%	Musc	Pain in joint/bones, 12.7%	Musc
2	Pain in back/neck, 13.6	Musc	Pain in back/neck, 9.5	Musc
3	Ringing in ears, 9.1	Eye/ear	Fatigue/no energy/lack of pep, 7.7	Gen
4	Pain/etc. in face/arm/leg[j], 5.8	Musc	Pain/etc. in face/arm/leg, 7.5	Musc
5	Skin rash, 4.2	Skin	Swollen leg/foot/ankle, 6.4	Musc
6	Feeling nervous/tense, 4.1	Psych	Headache or migraine, 4.9	Nerv
7	Swollen leg/foot/ankle, 4.0	Musc	Allergy symptoms, 4.8	Resp
8	Irregular heartbeat, 3.6	Circ	Shortness of breath, 3.9	Resp
9	Fatigue/no energy/lack of pep, 3.3	Gen	Cough, 3.5	Resp
10	Trouble seeing, even w/ glasses; Allergy symptoms, 3.2 (N=910 symptoms reported)	Eye/ear, Resp	Sore throat or hoarseness, 3.1 (N=1855)	Resp

d. The Detroit study focused on physical symptoms. Respondents rarely reported emotional ones such as anxiety or depression, but they did frequently report stress-related symptoms such as tension and nervousness. These physically felt, but psychologically toned, symptoms are classified in the Psychological group.

e. The Needs of the Elderly Study had a probability sample of older adult (ages 60+, 1982) residents of the Detroit suburb of Southfield. During NES III (1984), respondents kept health diaries for a total of 6 weeks (in three separate time segments). Data shown here are from the first 2-week segment. Data are not adjusted for dropout, which occurred for only several cases.

f. Ranks for two age groups, 62-74 and 75+, are very similar to the overall (62+) shown here; available from author.

g. Each symptom's major group is shown on the right.

h. The word trouble refers to pain, stiffness, aching, soreness, swelling, cramps, etc., in the location named.

i. Ranks based on "percent of people with symptom anytime in 2 weeks" are similar to those here.

j. Pain/weakness/numbness.

Specific symptoms (Table 2.11, bottom panel) also show the predominance of musculoskeletal problems for older men and women. General symptoms of overall pain, fatigue, and tension are also very visible in their lists. In middle ages (45-64), headache takes rank 1, and respiratory symptoms are common. Both descend sharply in importance with age, superseded by pain in numerous body sites.

The kinds of symptoms that bother middle-aged men and women are very similar; the same holds for older people. But symptoms are much more frequent for women at all ages (Table 2.12) (except Detroit, 65+).[13,14] Once again, we have evidence of the greater illness burden day by day, year by year, in women's lives than in men's.

TABLE 2.12 Rates of Daily Symptoms, for Age-Sex Groups

(Based on prospective health diaries. Two community studies.)

Detroit	Men			Women		
	18-44	45-64	65+	18-44	45-64	65+
	(Averages in 6 Weeks)					
No. symptomatic days	13.1	11.2	17.9	17.6	18.5	18.1
No. syndromes of symptoms[a]	16.3	13.0	30.9	25.8	28.7	31.0
No. specific symptoms	25.0	17.7	46.7	41.6	44.6	40.6

Southfield	Men			Women		
	62-74	75+	All 62+	62-74	75+	All 62+
	(Average in 2 Weeks)					
No. specific symptoms	15.0	15.9	15.2	18.2	29.6	22.6

SOURCE: Health in Detroit Study, 1978; Needs of the Elderly Study III, 1984. Brief descriptions of the studies are in Table 2.11 footnotes.

Self-Rated Health

Somehow, people add it all up. Considering their symptom experiences in the recent past, their longer-term chronic problems, and maybe even their beliefs about future prospects, people arrive at an overall evaluation of their health. The sex differences here are telling: Men are more likely to report the poles of health—excellent or poor—while women concentrate on more moderate responses—very good, good, fair (Table 2.13). Even as health evaluations drift downward with age, men are more likely to report *excellent* health than women. Things are not so certain for the other pole; men's excess of *poor* health certainly persists to age 75. Does it disappear after that, as the 1986 data suggest? Do elderly women drift toward fair/poor evaluations and men take over the moderate ones? Earlier data for 1978, however, show the persistence of more "poor" evaluations by men even at advanced ages (Ries, 1983; see also Whites in Havlik et al., 1987: Table 13). We tend to believe the basic pattern persists at all ages. Such a pattern reflects the differences noted throughout this section: Women are more bothered by symptoms, but realize that their problems are largely non-life-threatening. By contrast, men with "killer" conditions recognize the threat, while those thankfully free of such problems have little else going wrong.

TABLE 2.13 Self-Rated Health Status, for Age-Sex Groups, 1985 and 1986, United States

| | *(Percent Distribution)[a]* | | | | |
	Excellent	*Very Good*	*Good*	*Fair*	*Poor*
1985					
Male					
25-44	46.3	29.5	18.6	4.3	1.3
45-64	29.5	25.4	27.1	11.4	6.6
65+	16.5	19.7	31.4	21.3	11.1
Female					
25-44	38.6	30.9	23.4	5.6	1.5
45-64	24.6	25.2	31.1	13.4	5.7
65+	15.4	20.6	33.3	21.7	9.0
Sex Difference (F-M)					
25-44	− 7.7	1.4	4.8	1.3	0.2
45-64	− 4.9	− 0.2	4.0	2.0	− 0.9
65+	− 1.1	0.9	1.9	0.4	− 2.1
1986					
Male					
45-54	35.8	27.2	24.3	8.8	3.9
55-64	22.6	24.0	31.1	14.1	8.2
65-74	18.2	22.2	32.5	18.0	9.1
75-84	13.7	19.7	32.5	23.2	10.9
85+	19.9	20.9	29.8	18.6	10.8*
Female					
45-54	28.6	28.3	28.3	10.7	4.1
55-64	19.4	24.6	33.1	15.2	7.7
65-74	16.4	21.0	34.8	19.8	8.0
75-84	15.2	19.3	32.1	21.1	12.3
85+	16.1	20.3	28.3	22.3	13.0
Sex Difference (F-M)					
45-54	− 7.2	1.1	4.0	1.9	0.2
55-64	− 3.2	0.6	2.0	1.1	− 0.5
65-74	− 1.8	− 1.2	2.3	1.8	− 1.1
75-84	1.5	− 2.9	− 0.4	− 2.1	1.4
85+	− 3.8	− 0.6	− 1.5	3.7	2.2*

SOURCE: For 1985: National Health Interview Survey, 1985. Data in *Vital and Health Statistics*, Series 10, No. 160, (DHHS Publ. No. [PHS] 86-1588), Table 70. For 1986: Unpublished estimates for the National Health Interview Survey, 1986, provided by the National Center for Health Statistics.

* High relative standard error (over 30%) for rate.

a. Adds to 100.0 in each row.

Hypotheses About Health

Federal surveys provide these statistics on health status: (a) prevalence rates of chronic conditions taken one at a time, and (b) the global summary, self-rated health. The information contained in these is quite limited: Prevalence rates say nothing about the combinations of health problems people have, the timing or sequence of their entry into people's lives, or their symptomatic status. Self-rated health reveals no details about the components making up that evaluation.

The issues of *incidence, duration, comorbidity,* and *severity* are all fundamental to knowing the state of health among older women and men. We state some hypotheses about these "hidden dimensions" that need scientific research:

1. Women have higher incidence rates for most nonfatal diseases. With the reasonable assumption that chronic diseases are permanent (once acquired, always present to some degree), this hypothesis is implied, albeit imperfectly, by higher prevalence rates for women at all ages. It is difficult to see why women may be more vulnerable to this great variety of conditions, whose causal factors certainly vary. No global risk factors should be sought, but instead the specific risks that lie behind each condition.

2. Higher incidence plus longer lifetimes mean that women typically live with nonfatal conditions more total years than do men. Furthermore, women's lower incidence of fatal diseases may be compromised by their spending more years enduring the diseases after onset; thus, a scenario of "later but longer."

3. Women have more chronic health problems, on average, that do men. Chance alone (applying incidence rates independently) will cause women to have more comorbidity. If non-chance factors are also operating for women, such as heightened vulnerability to new diseases when others already exist, this further elevates their likelihood of comorbidity.

4. Are women's nonfatal conditions more often symptomatic and medically advanced that men's? We state no hypotheses about sex differences in botheration and progression of these diseases; both aspects must be considered in assessing severity. With respect to fatal diseases, it is reasonable to anticipate that women tend to have milder or less medically advanced conditions (see Waldron, 1983b for some evidence on the issue).

These hypotheses can be stated from the perspective of men. We hypothesize that middle-aged and older men have (1) typically lower incidence rates for nonfatal chronic diseases, and higher incidence rates for most fatal ones; (2) shorter duration of fatal and nonfatal conditions they develop; (3) fewer total chronic problems; and (4) generally more advanced fatal conditions.

(Note: These hypotheses use the terms condition and disease with care. Conditions encompass both disease and structural/sensory impairment. Impairments actually ensue from disease or injury. Although we can bring them into some of the hypotheses, we must always recognize that they are one step beyond disease itself, and that understanding sex differentials in risks of disease and injury is a prior step to understanding the impairment differentials.)

No stereotypes are intended in these hypotheses. Sex differences reveal tendencies, not absolutes, and they exist within the context of great similarity for the sexes. *Older men and women encounter largely the same types of health problems*; their lists of leading conditions and symptoms are more similar than different. *But the paces differ, with fatal conditions entering men's lives earlier and nonfatal ones, especially arthritis, entering women's lives earlier.* Thus, what distinguishes men and women most is frequencies (rates), not types of problems (ranks).

REFERENCES: For further reading on sex differences in health for middle-aged and older people, see Collins, 1986; Haug, Ford, & Sheafor, 1985; Hing, Kovar, & Rice, 1983; Mechanic, 1976; Nathanson, 1977; Nathanson & Lorenz, 1982; Verbrugge, 1976b, 1982, 1983, 1984a, 1985a, 1985b; Verbrugge & Wingard, 1987; Waldron, 1983b; Wingard, 1984.

DISABILITY

The Impacts of Disease

Chronic health problems can have great impact on a person's physical and social functioning, such as the ability to walk, enter or exit an automobile, or reach for objects, and the ability to dress oneself, go shopping, embroider, play tennis, or perform a paid job. A simple scheme for delineating the impacts of disease has been developed (World Health Organization, 1980) (Figure 2.2).[15] *Impairment* refers to manifestations of disease/injury at particular body sites such as

Figure 2.2 Conceptual Scheme for Disease Impact

DISEASE, INJURY,→ OR CONGENITAL MALFORMATION	IMPAIRMENT ⟶	DISABILITY ⟶	HANDICAP
(the intrinsic pathology or disorder)	(loss or abnormality of physiological, anatomical, or psychological structure/function)	(tasks of everyday life that a person cannot do alone or can do alone but with difficulty)(also often includes difficulties in basic physical movements/strength and mobility)	(disadvantages with respect to social roles and physical environment)

SOURCE: World Health Organization (1980).

mechanical impairment of shoulder, blind in one eye, shortness of breath. *Disability* refers to activities of daily and social life, such as personal care and household management tasks, and ability to perform job, family, and social roles. It can also include dysfunctions in physical abilities, such as limited endurance, strength, and range of motion in various body sites. Thus, there are two classes of disability: *physical disability* for the local dysfunctions and *social disability* for dysfunctions in "whole" tasks of living. *Handicap* concerns the interaction between person and environment and refers to restricted opportunities to accomplish desired goals and tasks. The scheme draws a typical time sequence, but at any given point, the preceding stages are not necessary or sufficient. All the paths are probabilities, and whether the outcomes actually happen to a person depends on the severity and type of problem at each stage and on medical and social efforts aimed at the pathways.

To date, health surveys have focused on *social disability*, especially on three kinds: personal care tasks (called activities of daily living, or ADL), household management tasks (called instrumental activities of daily living, or IADL), and major productive role (job, housework). In contrast, less is known about basic *physical disabilities*, such as musculoskeletal and cardiopulmonary capabilities, in the population. This is being remedied in several current population health surveys. Skeletal and sensory *impairments* are regularly measured in federal surveys like the National Health Interview Survey (NHIS)—see the prior section of this chapter. But others in the WHO scheme (intellectual, psychological, chronic visceral symptoms, disfigurement, etc.) are less often ascertained. *Handicap* is an elusive concept, very difficult to measure in respondent-based interviews. It is usually left to policy discussion rather than to empirical measurement.

This section concentrates on social disability, with some brief statements on physical disability.

Social Disability

There are two basic approaches to measuring social disability: one is epidemiological, the other policy oriented. The first focuses on how much *difficulty* a person has doing an activity on his/her own (without special aids or personal assistance) and whether that difficulty is due to a health problem. For ADL, actual performance ("do you do X by yourself . . . ?") is queried. For IADL, potential performance ("can/could you do X by yourself . . . ?") is preferred. Asking "do you do X" is not very informative here, since many people do not do household tasks (another family member or paid individual does) for reasons other than health. For social roles, complete or partial inability to perform them is queried. In sum, when asking about difficulty, the aim is to understand how health problems affect social capabilities. This is called the epidemiology of disability.[16] The second approach focuses on independence vs. *dependence*; namely, whether someone receives help from another person for a personal or household task due to a health problem. Typically, people are asked about receipt of help ("do you receive help from another person in X . . . ?"), rather than need for it ("do you need help from another person . . . ?"). Dependency rates are useful for making projections of long-term care needs. The ultimate aim is to make good estimates of current and future health services needs, and to craft appropriate public policies.

Because this chapter is about the state of health of men and women, rather than their use of or needs for health services, we will emphasize difficulty rates rather than dependency rates, when the data permit. We begin with activities of daily life (ADL and IADL) and then social roles.

Abilities to eat, transfer (get in and out of both a bed and chair), toilet (get to and use the toilet), dress and bathe are essential for human self-care.[17] In childhood these ADL skills are usually acquired in the order stated: eating first (the simplest of the activities), bathing last (the most complex). When chronic diseases impede self-care, difficulty and dependency tend to happen in the reverse sequence: loss of bathing abilities first, and eating last. IADLs concern ability to manage a household in contemporary society, or stated in another manner, to live independently in the modern setting. Abilities deemed essential are to shop for personal items, prepare one's own meals, manage one's own money, use the telephone, and do light housework. Whether these follow a typical sequence of developmental gain, or of loss in face of physical/mental disease, is not known now.[18] (IADL abilities are greatly affected by mental as well as physical disease.) But activities away from home usually place more demands on an individual than those at home and thus are almost certainly the "first to go."

Relatively few people living in the community (the noninstitutional population) have ADL and IADL problems. Rates increase with age, but are small until age 85+ for both sexes (Table 2.14).[19] Women are more likely to have difficulty doing all the activities, except telephone use and eating. The sex differences tend to get larger as age increases; thus, females' "extra" troubles are more obvious. The sizeable differences from age 85 onward partly reflect women's older average age in that span and, most likely, a real expansion in age-specific differences.

What constitutes a person's major activity, or productive role, is affected by age and sex. In middle ages, work (job) or household care are the usual principal activities, with the former typical for men, and either for women. In older ages, "retirement" from any major role is still expected (a pernicious piece of culture that one hopes will be abandoned), and no particular activities are prescribed for either sex. Work, housework, and other activities vary in their levels of physical demand and, thus, in people's chances of being limited when in poor health. This causes plenty of trouble in interpreting rates of disability for "major activity."

Table 2.15 shows limitation rates from three perspectives: major activity, work, and ADL/IADL. Readers are encouraged to read the footnotes for Table 2.15 to see the exact questions now used in the National Health Interview Survey.[20]

1. *Limitations in major activity* do not rise steadily with age because the question changes at age 70. Dependency (needing assistance from others) is a much "stronger" criterion of disability than difficulty doing job/housekeeping, and rates plummet as they cross from the lesser to greater criterion. Within each definition, disability does rise with age (from 45-64 to 65-69; then from 70-74 to 85+).[21]

   a. At *mild* levels (secondary activities), women are more likely disabled up to age 70. The higher rates for men thereafter certainly occur because some men think of their inability to work at a job!

TABLE 2.14 Difficulty in Performing Personal Care and Household Management Tasks, by Age-Sex Groups, United States, 1984.

Personal Care (ADL)[b]	*(Percent of Persons Who Have Difficulty Performing the Activity)[a]*				
	Bathe	*Dress*	*Transfer*	*Toilet*	*Eat*
Male					
65-74	5.7	4.4	4.8	2.4	1.5
75-84	9.2	7.3	6.0	3.6	2.5
85+	23.1	14.1	12.7	10.0	4.3
Female					
65-74	6.9	4.2	7.0	2.7	0.9
75-84	14.2	7.7	11.2	6.5	2.4
85+	30.1	17.7	22.2	15.9	4.4
Sex Difference (F-M)					
65-74	1.2	− 0.2	2.2	0.3	− 0.6
75-84	5.0	0.4	5.2	2.9	− 0.1
85+	7.0	3.6	9.5	5.9	0.1

Household Management (IADL)[c]	*Shop*	*Light Housework*	*Prepare Meals*	*Manage Money*	*Use Telephone*
Male					
65-74	4.6	3.5	3.0	2.8	3.5
75-84	9.6	6.2	6.0	5.4	7.9
85+	26.8	15.2	18.5	19.0	18.4
Female					
65-74	7.8	5.0	4.8	1.8	2.0
75-84	18.4	10.5	10.5	6.8	4.8
85+	41.6	27.4	29.5	26.2	17.1
Sex Difference (F-M)					
65-74	3.2	1.5	1.8	− 1.0	− 1.5
75-84	8.8	4.3	4.5	1.4	− 3.1
85+	14.8	12.1	11.0	7.2	− 1.3

SOURCE: Supplement on Aging, National Health Interview Survey, 1984. Derived from Dawson et al. (1987).

a. For ADL: "by yourself and without using special equipment." For IADL: "by yourself." For both, the difficulty must by stated as due to a health or physical problem.

b. The items are arranged from highest to lowest rates (for Both Sexes, 65+). Dependency (having personal assistance) rates follow the same order, at lower levels. Studies of institutional residents often find a switch for transfer and toilet, with higher dependency for toileting (Katz and Akpom, 1976).

c. The items are arranged from highest to lowest rates (for Both Sexes, 65+).

b. Women are more disabled in *moderate* (kind/amount) ways than men, regardless of the question.

c. Middle-aged men report complete inability to do their major activity more often. This partly reflects greater demands that jobs other than housekeeping place on people; a larger percentage of men than women these ages view their job as their major activity. At very elderly ages, *severe* disability (ADL dependence) is more prevalent among women.[22]

Interpretations are simpler when a single activity is considered.

2. *Work limitations* rise with age for both men and women (Table 2.15). The sex differences are not very big; rates are usually a little higher for men. If women's jobs tend to be less physically taxing than men's, then even these differences have ambiguous meaning. Apart from that, research has shown that women with health-related job limitations quit the labor force more readily than comparably ill men; once this happens, women function reasonably well in their revised major activity, housekeeping (in the top panel, the percent unable is much lower for them than men).

3. *ADL and IADL limitations* rise with age for both sexes.[23] At all ages, women are more likely than men to have IADL dependency, and at advanced ages ADL dependency.

Can the results be summarized? We acknowledge first that their variety is intentional. The shifting standards for work vs. housekeeping, type of job, and activities of daily living vs. productive roles are conscious ones. Still, socially speaking, the data indicate that more women suffer mild and moderate kinds of disability at all ages. (We take the prerogative to reinterpret the secondary activity data for men ages 70+.) The sexes are quite similar for severe personal care problems until very elderly ages, when women show more disability. More trouble for men shows up in major activity and work limitations, mainly because many women have less physically demanding roles (housework and even types of jobs).

Why are women more likely to be disabled, especially in moderate ways? Why do men equal or surpass them in severe disability until very old ages? The answers are both medical (the different kinds of health problems men and women have) and social (how those problems interact with role demands, and the success of medical and personal therapy and rehabilitation). Medically speaking, one plausible reason for women's higher disability prevalence is simply their higher illness and

TABLE 2.15 Rates of Social Disability (Activity, Work, and IADL/ADL Limitations), by Age-Sex Groups, 1983-85, United States

Activity Limitation[b]	*(Percent Distribution)*[a]			
	Not Limited in Activity	*·Limited in Secondary Activity Only*	*Limited in Kind/Amount of Major Activity*	*Unable to Perform Major Activity*
Men				
45-64	77.1 }74.2	4.2 } 4.3	7.8 } 8.5	10.9 }13.1
65-69	59.0	4.8	11.9	24.3
70-74	65.6 }63.6	24.0 }22.2	6.3 } 8.5	4.1 } 5.7
75-84	61.7	20.4	10.6	7.3
85+	44.6	16.6	21.6	17.2
Women				
45-64	75.5 }72.9	7.2 } 7.9	11.1 }12.3	6.2 } 6.9
65-69	60.9	11.1	17.8	10.2
70-74	67.1 }62.5	17.9 }17.0	10.9 }14.3	4.1 } 6.1
75-84	58.8	16.3	17.1	7.8
85+	39.6	10.9	29.5	20.0
Sex Difference (F-M)				
45-64	– 1.6	3.0	3.3	– 4.7
65-69	1.9	6.3	5.9	–14.1
70-74	1.5	– 6.1	4.6	0.0
75-84	– 2.9	– 4.1	6.5	0.5
85+	– 5.0	– 5.7	7.9	2.8

Work Limitation[c]	*Not Limited in Work Activity*	*Limited in Kind/Amount of Work*	*Unable to Work*
Men			
45-64	81.3	7.6	11.1
65-69	63.7	11.5	14.8
Women			
45-64	81.0	6.6	12.4
65-69	69.0	8.4	12.6
Sex Difference (F-M)			
45-64	– 0.3	– 1.0	1.3
65-69	5.3	– 3.1	– 2.2

(*continued*)

TABLE 2.15 Continued

IADL/ADL Limitation[d]	Not Limited in IADL/ADL	Limited in IADL Only	Limited in ADL (Needs Assistance)
Men			
45-64	96.5 }96.0	2.3 } 2.6	1.2 } 1.4
65-69	93.4	4.0	2.6
70-74	89.6 }85.8	6.3 } 8.5	4.1 } 5.7
75-84	82.1	10.6	7.3
85+	61.2	21.6	17.2
Women			
45-64	94.9 }94.2	3.9 } 4.4	1.2 } 1.4
65-69	91.1	6.6	2.3
70-74	85.0 }79.5	10.9 }14.3	4.1 } 6.1
75-84	75.1	17.1	7.8
85+	50.5	29.5	20.0
Sex Difference (F-M)			
45-64	− 1.6	1.6	0.0
65-69	− 2.3	2.6	− 0.3
70-74	− 4.6	4.6	0.0
75-84	− 7.0	6.5	0.5
85+	−10.7	7.9	2.8

SOURCE: National Health Interview Survey, 1983-85. Derived from data in LaPlante (1988: Tables 2,3,4).

a. Adds to 100.0 in each row.

b. For ages 45-69, major activity is work (job) or keeping house. For ages 70+, "unable" means needs assistance in ADL; "limited in kind or amount of major activity" means needs assistance in IADL only. For all ages 45+, secondary activity limitation is queried only if no major activity limitation exists. People keeping house who report work limitation (see next footnote) automatically are counted as having secondary activity limitation. Overall, limitations are counted only if due to an impairment or health problem.

c. All people ages 45-69 are asked about their ability to work at a job or business.

d. Persons ages 45-69 with activity limitation, and all persons ages 60+, are asked about ADL assistance and (if none) IADL assistance. The two questions asked in NHIS are: "Because of any impairment or health problem, does (NAME) need the help of other persons in personal care needs, such as eating, bathing, dressing, or getting around this house?", ". . . need the help of other persons in handling routine needs, such as everyday household chores, doing necessary business, shopping, or getting around for other purposes?" People with ADL dependency are assumed to have IADL dependency as well, but this is not queried directly.

symptom rates. One reason for men's equally severe disability (ADL) until advanced ages may be earlier and faster-paced experience of fatal diseases. These statements remain to be tested, and they are certainly only one piece of the whole story.

Physical Disability

How do men and women fare for walking (gross mobility), motions such as reaching or stooping, and strength for lifting things? Now we strip away social context and compare the sexes' performance in uniform activities. In surveys to date, this is usually done by interviewers asking about standard tasks, but there is growing commitment to getting actual observations of performance during the interview.

The data available show that women have higher rates of all physical disabilities, especially tasks requiring strength or involving the lower extremities. The latter is certainly influenced by their higher arthritis rates.

Leading Limiting Conditions

Just as we have considered leading causes of death and leading chronic conditions, let us determine the leading causes of limitation. Which chronic conditions are most limiting? This is really two questions: (1) What proportion of the population is limited by X? This *overall limitation* rate is a function of both condition prevalence (discussed in the prior section) and its "limiting potential," and (2) Given the presence of X, what is the likelihood of being limited by it? This is *limiting potential*, or the probability of dysfunction for people with the condition.[24]

Beginning with overall limitation rates: The foremost limiting conditions for middle-aged and older people are heart disease and arthritis (Table 2.16). Arthritis ranks first for women, and heart disease for men. Arthritis limits activities for 5.9 percent of women at ages 45-64 and 14.3 percent at 65+. Heart disease limits activities for 5.9 percent of men at ages 45-64 and 13.5 percent at 65+. Besides these, the lists of leading limiters are filled with musculoskeletal and circulatory problems of many kinds, for both age groups and both sexes. Some high-prevalence conditions are completely absent, such as chronic sinusitis, tinnitus, hay fever, and (almost absent) hearing impairments. And some low-prevalence conditions, which do not surface at all in Table 2.8, show up as significant limiters; examples are malignant neoplasms, mental problems, and paralysis.[25]

TABLE 2.16 Leading Limiting Chronic Conditions, for Age-Sex Groups, United States, 1979-80

(Conditions Causing Limitation in Major or Secondary Activity, per 1,000 Population. Average Annual Rate.)[a,b]

MEN, 45-64	WOMEN, 45-64
1 Diseases of heart, 59.4	Arthritis, 59.0
2 Arthritis, 36.2	Diseases of heart, 38.2
3 High blood pressure, 26.5	High blood pressure, 33.9
4 Def./orth. impairment[c]-back/spine, 25.1	Def./orth. impair.-back/spine, 22.0
5 Other musculoskeletal disorders[d], 23.9	Other musculoskel. disorders. 21.4
6 Def./orth. impairment-lower extrem., 20.4	Diabetes,17.2
7 Diabetes, 14.8	Def./orth. imp.-lower extrem.,13.9
8 Atherosclerosis, 14.1	Atherosclerosis, 9.8
9 Emphysema, 13.4	Malignant neoplasms, 9.6
10 Visual impairments, 8.9	Asthma, 8.4
11 Other respiratory disease[e], 8.5	Mental symptoms, 7.9
12 Paralysis, 8.0	Other digestive diseases, 6.5
13 Def./orth. imp.-upper extrem., 7.7	Visual impairment, 6.4
14 Other digestive diseases[f], 7.5	Other impairments[g], 5.9
15 Hernia of abdominal cavity, 7.1	Emphysema, 5.3

MEN, 65+	WOMEN, 65+
1 Diseases of heart, 135.0	Arthritis, 143.1
2 Arthritis, 82.4	Diseases of heart, 93.2
3 High blood pressure, 46.5	High blood pressure, 65.3
4 Emphysema, 39.0	Diabetes, 30.7
5 Atherosclerosis, 34.9	Def./orth. imp.-lower extrem., 29.7
6 Visual impairments, 31.1	Visual impairments, 29.6
7 Diabetes, 27.7	Atherosclerosis, 25.5
8 Def./orth. imp.-lower extrem., 25.1	Def./orth. imp.-back/spine, 20.5
9 Cerebrovascular disease, 24.5	Other musculoskel. disorders, 17.2
10 Paralysis, 21.0	Cerebrovascular disease, 15.0
11 Other musculoskeletal disorders, 18.4	Paralysis, 12.4
12 Def./orth. impairment-back/spine, 18.0	Malignant neoplasms, 12.4
13 Malignant neoplasms, 17.7	Other digestive diseases, 11.4
14 Other respiratory diseases, 17.3	Hearing impairments, 11.4
15 Hearing impairments, 14.3	Hernia of abdominal cavity, 9.2

SOURCE: Calculated from unpublished data for the National Health Interview Survey, 1979-80, provided by the National Center for Health Statistics. A table for ages 45-69, 70-84, 85+ based on 1983-85 data is available on request. This table appears in Verbrugge (1987) with detailed notes.

a. There are 53 titles, which encompass all chronic conditions in the International Classification of Diseases. All rates shown here have low sampling error (relative standard error 30% or less).

b. Major activity is job or housekeeping; secondary activities are clubs, shopping, church attendance, etc. In 1979-80, for major activity: All men were asked about job; women whose usual activity was housekeeping were asked about housework limitations; women whose usual activity was job, retired, or something else were asked about job. This approach was changed in 1982; the current one is described in Table 2.15, footnote b.

c. Deformity or orthopedic impairment. Absence/paralysis is not included.

d. Excludes arthritis.

e. Excludes chronic bronchitis, emphysema, asthma, hay fever without asthma, and chronic sinusitis.

f. Excludes ulcer of stomach/duodenum, hernia of abdominal cavity, and gallbladder diseases.

g. Excludes back/spine, upper extremity, lower extremity, and multiple impairments.

TABLE 2.17 Comparing Prevalence and Activity Limitations from Chronic Conditions

(21 titles are ranked for prevalence, limitation, and limiting potential.
Rank 1 is highest value, and Rank 21 is lowest.)[a]

	Men 45-69			Men 70-84			Men 85+		
	Prev.	*Lim.*	*Lim. Pot.*	*Prev.*	*Lim.*	*Lim. Pot*	*Prev.*	*Lim.*	*Lim. Pot.*
Arthritis	5	2	13	2	3	11	3	3	9
Intervertebral disc	13	8	3	18	17	7	16*	18*	15
Other skin/musc. cond.	4	14	19	6	14	19	7	15*	18
Absence/paralysis	12	11	15	10	8	6	11	5	3
Back impairments	9	5	11	14	15	10	10	15*	12
Lower extrem. imp.	10	6	10	15	10	4	13*	6	1
Oth.orthoped. imp.	16	17	9	17	19	12	17*	17*	5
Eye/ear diseases/imp.	2	4	18	1	2	14	1	1	11
Digestive cond.	6	10	17	7	11	17	5	9	17
Heart diseases	7	1	7	4	1	7	2	2	10
Hypertension	3	3	14	5	4	15	6	11*	16
Cerebrovas.disease	17	15	6	12	5	2	9	6	7
Other circulatory cond.	8	12	16	8	7	16	4	4	14
Asthma	15	18	12	16	18	13	18	18*	6
Emphysema	14	9	2	11	6	3	15	13*	3
Other respiratory cond.[b]	1	13	20	3	12	18	8	8	13
Diabetes	11	7	8	9	9	9	12	12*	8
Mental illness	na	19	na	na	20	na	na	18*	na
Mental retardation	20*	21	1	20*	21*	1	—	21*	—
Nervous system cond.[c]	18	15	5	19	13	na	18*	14*	na
Cancer, all sites[d]	19	20	4	13	16	5	14*	9	2

SOURCE: National Health Interview Survey, 1983-85. Calculated by author from data in LaPlante (1988: Tables 1,6B).

na Cannot be estimated (no numerator counts for mental illness; implausible ratio over 1.00 for nervous system cond.).

* High sampling error (relative standard error > 30%).

— Zero cases in sample.

a. The 21 titles cover the great majority of limiting chronic conditions (89% of all mentions). This table is based on all mentions; results for main cause are available from author. Due to space constraints, the calculated rates for prevalence, limitation, and limiting potential are not shown (available from author); only their ranks are shown. (Prevalence rate is conditions per 1,000 pop. Limitation rate is conditions causing major or secondary activity limitation per 1,000 pop. Limiting potential is the ratio of limitation rate to prevalence rate.) Tied ranks (in a column) occur when the population estimates of prevalence/limitation for the several conditions are identical, or when their limiting potential ratios are identical. When ties occur, the next rank number (n+1) is skipped and the count resumes at n+2. Maximum rank possible for prevalence and limiting potential is 20, due to n.a. for Mental Illness prevalence in population.

(continued)

TABLE 2.17 Continued

Women 45-69			Women 70-84			Women 85+		
Prev.	*Lim.*	Lim. Pot.	*Prev.*	Lim.	*Lim. Pot.*	*Prev.*	Lim.	*Lim. Pot.*
2	1	13	2	1	12	2	2	6
14	10	3	17	19	8	18*	18*	2
3	8	19	5	9	19	2	9	17
15	16	8	12	11	7	14	11	3
9	6	12	9	12	14	11	12	13
12	9	10	11	6	4	9	4	1
17	19	7	16	18	13	15	15	9
6	5	16	1	3	16	1	1	11
5	7	17	4	7	18	4	8	16
8	3	9	7	2	9	6	3	5
4	2	15	3	4	15	5	5	15
18	20	6	12	10	5	10	7	4
7	11	18	8	8	17	7	6	14
13	13	11	15	17	10	16*	18*	12
19	18	2	19	16	2	19*	20*	8
1	15	20	6	15	20	8	16*	18
10	4	5	10	5	3	12	10	7
na	17	na	na	20	na	na	17*	na
20*	21	1	20*	21*	11	—	21*	—
11	12	14	18	14	na	17*	12	na
16	14	4	14	13	6	13	14	10

b. Includes chronic sinusitis, a frequently reported condition in NHIS.

c. For nervous system conditions, the limitation rate covers more titles than the prevalence rate does. This inflates the limitation rate and limiting potential, and gives them more important (smaller-number) ranks than they merit. Caution is recommended.

d. For cancer, skin cancers of all kinds are included in the prevalence and limitation rates. (A very large fraction of skin cancers are nonmelanoma; they cause minimal disability and death.) This acts to deflate the limitation rate and limiting potential. Besides this, the limitation rate covers more titles than the prevalence rate does; and this acts to inflate those same items. The net effect of these two factors on, especially, limiting potential is unknown, but we suspect the first is more critical. We checked this by removing *all* skin cancers from the analysis: The prevalence ranks dropped in age-sex groups, the limitation ranks stayed about the same, and the limiting potential ranks zoomed up—often rising to first or second rank. In sum, readers can view the ranks for cancer's limiting potential as very conservative in Table 2.17.

The notion that prevalence and limitation are not necessarily concordant is borne out in Table 2.17. For 21 titles, covering the majority of limiting chronic conditions, we show ranks for prevalence, overall limitation, and limiting potential.[26] Three clear results appear.

TABLE 2.18 Comparing Prevalence and IADL/ADL Limitation from Chronic Conditions

(21 titles are ranked for prevalence, limitation, and limiting potential.
Rank 1 is highest value, and Rank 21 is lowest.)[a]

	Men 70+			Women 70+		
	Prev.	Lim.	*Lim. Pot.*	*Prev.*	Lim.	*Lim. Pot.*
Arthritis	2	3	12	2	1	11
Intervertebral disc disorders	18	19*	10	17	20	12
Other skin/musculoskel. cond.	7	15	20	5	10	19
Absence/paralysis	10	5	5	13	11	8
Back impairments	13	17	14	9	14	15
Lower extremity imp.	14	10	4	11	6	4
Other orthopedic imp.	17	20*	13	15	17	10
Eye/ear diseases/imp.	1	1	11	1	2	14
Digestive conditions	6	13	18	4	9	18
Heart diseases	3	2	9	7	3	9
Hypertension	5	6	17	3	4	16
Cerebrovascular disease	11	4	3	12	8	3
Other circulatory conditions	8	8	16	8	7	17
Asthma	16	18	15	16	19	13
Emphysema	12	9	6	19	16	2
Other respiratory conditions	4	14	19	6	15	20
Diabetes	9	7	8	10	5	6
Mental illness	na	16	na	na	18	na
Mental retardation	20*	21*	1	20*	21*	5
Nervous system cond.	19	11	2	18	12	1
Cancer, all sites	15	12	7	14	13	7

SOURCE: National Health Interview Survey, 1983-85. Calculated by author from data in LaPlante (1988: Tables 1,8B).

na Cannot be estimated (no prevalence estimates of mental illness are obtained in NHIS).

* High sampling error (relative standard error > 30%).

a. See footnote a. of Table 2.17. This table is based on all mentions; results for main cause are available from author. (The Limitation rate calculated for this table is conditions causing IADL/ADL dependence per 1,000 pop.)

1. The most prevalent diseases are not often disabling (limiting potential). Compare the first and third columns for arthritis, other skin/musculoskeletal, eye/ear, digestive, hypertension, other circulatory, and other respiratory (includes chronic sinusitis).

2. Low prevalence conditions are the most often disabling ones. See intervertebral disc disorders, absence/paralysis (ages 85+), lower extremity impairments (ages 70+), cerebrovascular disease (CVD), emphysema, mental retardation, and cancer.

3. Only a few diseases have quite consistent ranks for prevalence and limiting potential. These are back impairment, heart diseases, and diabetes.

With these two components—prevalence and limiting potential—we can now understand limitation rates in the second column. Arthritis, eye/ear, and hypertension are important in the aggregate because of sheer prevalence, while their disabling potential is quite low. Heart diseases' importance stems from moderately high prevalence combined with moderately high limiting potential.

Looking at dependence (needs for assistance in ADL or IADL), the same pattern of results appears (Table 2.18). Arthritis, eye/ear conditions, and (for women) hypertension are commonly stated as causes of dependence because of their very high prevalence; they have moderate or low limiting potential. CVD (men) ranks high because of its high disabling potential; its prevalence is only moderate. Heart diseases again rank high because of combined moderate/high prevalence and moderate limiting potential.

These results are consistent for both men and women: *the leading limiting conditions are similar for them, and so are their limiting potentials (chance of being disabled if one has the condition).* Once again, what distinguishes men and women most are rates of disability, not the kinds of problems that cause disability.

Active Life Expectancy

So far, all the data above show men's and women's status at a given time point (when interviewed). We need to insert some time perspective. How much disability do they endure over their whole lifetime? The notion of life expectancy, used in mortality analysis, can be adapted to answer this. Now we want to know the expected years of nondisabled life, not of life in toto. This is called "active life expectancy." Studies to date in the United States and several other developed countries show that women can expect several more years of nondisabled life than men can.[27] But they also have notably more total years of disability, on average, and thus the percent of their lifetimes spent disabled is greater than for men. This is true whether we look forward from birth (age 0) or from an older age, such as 65. For example, in a Massachusetts study, women at age 65 can expect 10.6 years of nondisabled life and men 9.3 (Katz et al., 1983). But the ratio of these numbers to life expectancy at age 65 ($10.6/19.5 = .54$ and $9.3/13.1 = .71$, respectively) is lower for women, indicating the larger fraction of late life they can expect to spend dependent or institutionalized. Thus, the lifetime toll of disability is much greater for women than for men, both in absolute and relative terms.

Disability Dynamics

Disability is not really a static feature, but can fluctuate over time and even disappear for good. These dynamics depend on medical status and interventions over time. Longitudinal data that track individuals' disability over time are becoming available. One study shows that (1) nondisabled women are more likely than men to become disabled over a time interval (higher disability incidence rates for women)[28] and (2) disabled men are slightly more likely to restore function over a time interval (Manton, 1988).

Institutionalization

Institutional residence can be counted as a form of disability, since it signals inability to function adequately in the community for medical or social reasons.[29] Institutional residence is more common for older women than older men (Table 2.19). And among residents, women typically have higher disability levels than men of similar age (Havlik et al., 1987: Table 59). For both sexes, institutions filter for more severely ill/disabled persons. Despite the tighter medical filter for women, their numbers still predominate in nursing and personal care homes. There is more to becoming a resident there than just health status.

REFERENCES: For discussions and data on ADL/IADL difficulty and dependence, see Dawson, Hendershot, & Fulton, 1987; Feller, 1983; Jette & Branch, 1981; Macken, 1986. Information on physical disability is in Foley, Berkman, Branch, Farmer, & Wallace, 1986; Haber, 1973 (for work-disabled people); Jette & Branch, 1981, 1984. Discussions of physical disability are in Branch & Meyers, 1987; Guralnik, 1987. For activity limitation and work disability, see LaPlante, 1988; Moss & Parsons, 1986; Nagi, 1976. Readers are cau-

TABLE 2.19 Residence in Nursing Homes and Personal Care Homes, by Age-Sex, 1985, United States

| | *(Institutional Residents per 1,000 Pop.)[a]* | | |
	Male	*Female*	*Sex Ratio (F/M)*
All Races[b]			
55-64	4.2	4.0	0.95
65-74	10.8	13.8	1.28
75-84	43.0	66.4	1.54
85+	145.7	250.1	1.72
White			
55-64	3.7	4.0	1.08
65-74	10.5	13.7	1.30
75-84	42.9	68.6	1.60
85+	150.4	258.0	1.72
Black			
55-64	9.3	4.2	0.45
65-74	14.5	16.0	1.10
75-84	45.6	45.1	0.99
85+	95.6	162.7	1.70

SOURCE: For All Races, ages 65+: *Health, United States, 1987*. (DHHS Publ. No. [PHS] 88-1232). National Center for Health Statistics, 1988. For All Races, ages 55-64: Unpublished data for the 1985 National Nursing Home Survey provided by the National Center for Health Statistics. For White and Black: *Vital and Health Statistics*, Series 3, No. 25, Table 5 (Havlik et al., 1987).

a. The denominator is the total population residing in the United States.
b. Includes white, black, other.

tioned that the terms used in disability research vary widely now and do not often match ours. We like the ones presented here, because they are clear and align closely with the WHO scheme.

The epidemiology of disability is discussed in Cornoni-Huntley et al., 1985; Haber, 1971; Manton & Soldo, 1985; Nagi, 1976; World Health Organization, 1984. Active life expectancy and disability dynamics are discussed in Branch, Katz, Kniepmann, & Papsidero, 1984; Crimmins & Saito, 1987; Katz et al., 1983; Robine et al., 1986; Rogers, Rogers, & Branch, in press; Wilkins & Adams, 1983a, 1983b. Data on institutional residence, a large issue only briefly treated in this chapter, are in Branch & Jette, 1982; Hing, 1981; Hing & Cypress, 1981, Liu & Manton, 1987.

TRAJECTORIES OF ILLNESS, DISABILITY, AND DEATH

Statistics usually give static views of health, indicating the percent or rate of people in a given state at a particular time. This disguises the truth of health: it is dynamic for individuals over their lives, with illness onsets and recoveries, insidious development of disability, and welcome returns to function. In late life, the dynamics become increasingly one-way. Chronic conditions (essentially "permanent" once they cross a diagnostic threshold) dominate health, and physiological ability to restore lost functions diminishes. The result is usually a net accretion of health and activity problems for individuals. But "net" is always different from "gross," and there is still plenty of action to watch in disease severity, symptoms, and specific disabilities.

A model trajectory of events over time is: clinical onset of chronic disease, followed later by problems in doing household management tasks and discretionary activities like hobbies and recreation, then securing assistance in IADLs, later difficulty in personal care activities, obtaining help with ADLs, leaving the community to reside in an institution, and death. This is portrayed in Figure 2.3, in the form of survival curves. These show proportions of population by age *not* in each state; thus, having "survived" the event.

Figure 2.3 presumes two things: that each state is *absorbing* ("once entered, never left") and that a *hierarchy* among states exists (people in a given state have all the "lesser" ones as well). These are convenient assumptions, but not completely true-to-life.

1. It is reasonable to view chronic morbidity as an absorbing state (this may change in the future if genuine cures for chronic problems are found). And death certainly is an absorbing one. But in between is disability in its various dimensions, and it is assuredly changeable. For example, people can go back and forth in IADL performance over several years; or they can return to community residence after an institutional stay.

2. Disability is also not hierarchical; people can have combinations of disability that do not match the model, such as dependence for an ADL but not for IADLs.

3. Last, it is important to recognize that most people follow the trajectory only partway, never reaching the far points of ADL dependence or institutionalization before they die.

In short, although aggregate rates are neatly ordered—with highest rates for illness, next for IADLs, then ADLs, institutionalization, and lowest for death—this is not proof of a single pathway for individuals.[30]

Figure 2.3 Model Survival Curves for Older Persons.

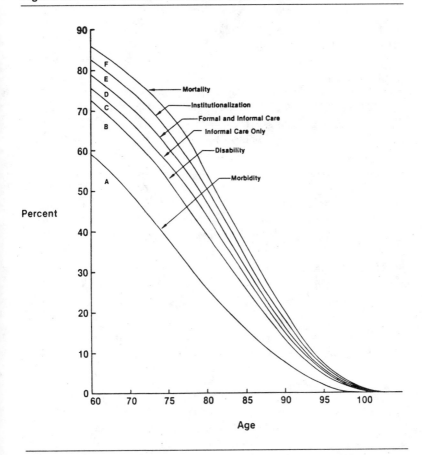

SOURCE: Soldo and Manton (1985).

Research in coming years will show us the "transition rates" among disability states in Figure 2.3. The simplifying assumptions of absorption and hierarchy will be abandoned to comply with real life. And research articles, such as this one, will cease to present mortality as their preface and put it in its proper place after discussions of health and disability.

Summing up what we know now about disability states (rates) and dynamics, *women's lives before the "finish line" of death are more filled with sickness and disability, a price paid for greater tendency to*

*acquire nonfatal chronic problems and for longer life; men cross that
line sooner, having suffered fewer years of trouble while alive.* Which
sex pays a higher price? There is no consensual way to answer this;
both prices are certainly high.

Why the paces of illness, disability, and death differ so greatly by
gender is a big issue. It is really multiple issues, since sex differences
go different directions in these domains and each needs it own explanation. These different directions—higher female morbidity and disability, but higher male mortality—do not imply an inherent
contradiction. Figure 2.3 helps us see the matter: Men simply reach
death sooner than women do, apparently skipping intermediate stages
of disability and/or spending less time in them. By contrast, women
tarry longer in the morbidity and disability zones. Thus, there are
differences in men's and women's pathways and paces along the model
trajectory, but no ultimate contradiction of what happens to them.
Research must aim at the sex differences *at each point*: Why do men's
and women's experiences here differ at all?

REFERENCES: Discussions of the juxtaposition of female excess
morbidity with male excess mortality are in Verbrugge, 1976a, 1988, in
press; Verbrugge & Wingard, 1987; Waldron, 1982.

THE POPULATION DYNAMICS OF GENDER AND AGING

The previous section addresses individual dynamics, the
probabilities of finding people in a state and of their movement from
one state to another. In this chapter, we have shown that age and sex
are important signals of different levels (rates) of health states, and
considered hypotheses and new data about transitions.

There is another, larger arena in which age and sex contribute to
health dynamics. Policymakers and health service providers are less
interested in individual trajectories over time than societal ones, namely, the total number of people with specific health problems and disabilities, now and in the future. Good forecasts hinge on knowing about
the future size of key population groups and their future rates of
illness/disability/mortality. We have amply discussed differential rates,
but not sex and age distribution of the population and its implications
for future needs.

The U.S. population is *aging*, thereby increasing the percent of
people at ages 65+. This general aging is accompanied by a special

feature called *aging-within-aging*: the 65+ group is itself aging, with increasing percents of older people being very old (85+). In addition, *feminization of the elderly* is occurring; that is, the percent of females is increasing in the 65+ group. Population aging and feminization of the elderly are not brand-new; aging has been a feature of our population dynamics throughout the twentieth century, and feminization has been ongoing since the 1930s. But the mortality declines launched around 1970 gave special impetus to aging-within-aging, since mortality gains have been concentrated at older ages.

Increasing percents of old (especially very old) people, and of old women rather than men, will change both the volume and composition of population health over the long run. If we assume that age-sex specific rates of illness/disability will stay the same, then these population dynamics will increase needs for medical and rehabilitation services, home assistance, and nursing beds and congregate housing. The increases will not be very large year by year, but will be noticeable over the long run of decades. Moreover, medical professionals' attention will necessarily shift toward chronic conditions that are symptomatic and disabling but not life-threatening, such as arthritis, incontinence, varicose veins, vision and hearing problems and digestive disorders.

The assumption of constant illness/disability rates is actually not a very good one. Morbidity and disability rates within age groups appear to be rising (Chapman, LaPlante, & Wilensky, 1986; Crimmins & Saito, 1987; Feldman, 1983; Rice & LaPlante, 1988; Verbrugge, 1984b, 1989; Yelin, in press). This fuels estimates of future needs still more.

REFERENCES: For population aging, see Rice & Feldman, 1983; Rosenwaike, 1985a, 1985b; Siegel, 1979; Siegel & Davidson, 1984; Taeuber, 1983; U. S. Senate Special Committee on Aging, 1986; Zopf, 1986. For discussions pertinent to this entire chapter that give other perspectives on aging and health, see Haynes & Feinleib, 1980; La-Londe, 1975; Manton & Soldo, 1985; Rice & LaPlante, 1988; Riley & Bond, 1983; Shanas, 1962, 1968; Soldo & Manton, 1985; Ward & Tobin, 1987.

CONCLUSION

It is a familiar picture in many families: Dad dies from cancer early in his retirement, and Mom lives to an advanced age but with incessant arthritis pain and circumscribed function. These pictures, writ large, become statistics of health, disability, and mortality. Individuals' own details get lost, but a more reliable view of life and death for middle-aged and older people emerges.

What starts as simple biology at birth rapidly gathers momentum and heft. Sex and age are the substrata for gender and aging, for continually becoming a man (woman) and becoming an older person. Differences in hormones, chromosomes, roles, life-styles, and attitudes lead to differential risks of illness for men and women, and also differential responses to illness. Differences in physiological repair and wear, accumulated extrinsic risks, social prescriptions for age groups, and lessons of experience cause differential risks of illness and disability for young, middle-aged, and older adults. The distribution of ages and sexes in a population determines health in the aggregate—the numbers of people with a given problem and the variety of problems present. Changes over time in individual-level risks for age-sex groups, and changes in population distribution, will alter aggregate problems and needs. Thus do age and sex wend their way through individual lifetimes and social change.

How long will the portrayal of age-sex differences in this chapter last? Specific *rates* will fluctuate from year to year, and may even change in systematic ways. Whatever causes those changes—social, environmental, cultural—will usually affect all age-sex groups, more in some and less in others, but usually parallel in direction. This means that group *differentials* are likely to be quite enduring, far less changeable than the rates underlying them. Our overall statements about women's tenacity despite pain and disability and men's too swift exit are likely to be as true several decades hence as now. The purpose of this chapter has been to point out those differences, not to answer why they exist. That is a large research agenda, which currently engages many scientists in fields stretching from entomology to demography.

Cloaked in biology and society, sex and age are heralds of health and dysfunction, declaring probabilities rather than certainties. Whatever those probabilities are, we shall always want them lower to keep people free of disease, disability, and death still longer. The challenge to policymakers is now to give as much serious attention to living as to dying, to the nonfatal conditions and difficulties in doing desired activities that compromise life's value in later life, especially for women. It is not just Dad's empty chair, but also Mom's grimace as she opens a car door, that matter.

NOTES

1. Nevertheless, the suddenness of the decline, whose onset is precisely dated at 1968, remains hard to explain. Most personal and medical inputs have slow, rather than swift, impact on population mortality.

2. There is instability from year to year in mortality rates at these high ages. We looked at changes from 1975 to 1980, 1981, 1982, . . ., 1985 for the 85+ group. Our text statements still hold: men at 85+ show rises for all of these time intervals, and women for most.

3. The increase in life endurancy, and the problems in obtaining gains in mortality among persons at 85+ due to very frail people (noted in a prior paragraph), are not contradictory. The overall declines in mortality at older ages leave us with a wider distribution of "robustness" than before, with a larger fraction extremely robust and a larger fraction extremely frail.

4. Sex differentials (All Causes) are largest for youths (ages 15-24) and young adults (25-34), then slowly narrow. At advanced ages (85+), the gap is about as large as in early childhood (see Metropolitan Life Insurance Co., 1988).

5. See also Verbrugge (1987) for age spans 17-44, 45-64, and 65+.

6. Smoking causes cardiovascular and respiratory diseases, and it accounts for roughly 50% of the male excess (Waldron, 1986b). External causes (accidents, suicide, homicide, other external) account for about 40% of the sex difference.

7. Further discussion, spanning all adult ages from 17-44 to 65+, is in Verbrugge (1987).

8. The term arthritis encompasses about one hundred specific diseases, whose primary manifestation is in the joints. Erosion of joint surfaces, inflammation of joint capsules, and structural changes in underlying bone prompt pain, swelling, and limited range of motion. The most common arthropathy is osteoarthritis, also called degenerative joint disease. It is frequently, often perpetually, symptomatic and progresses inexorably over a person's lifetime (onset is typically defined by x-ray evidence).

9. Are there any "women's health problems" and "men's health problems"? Only the few sex-specific conditions—feasible for one sex and not the other. These comprise reproductive problems such as menopausal symptoms and uterine/ovarian/cervical conditions for women, and benign prostatitis and cancer of prostate for men. One might include sex-dominant conditions—feasible for both sexes, but largely found in one. The clearest examples are osteoporosis, rheumatoid arthritis, stress incontinence, urinary tract infections, and breast cancer, all more common among women. A broad treatment of problems specific to or dominant in women is in Gold (1984).

10. The full list of titles with excess female rates is about twice the length shown in Table 9, top panel (available from author).

11. Only two national studies offer data on symptoms (Proprietary Association, 1984; Shanas, 1962). Both asked about symptoms retrospectively: for the past two weeks in the former, and the past four weeks in the latter. These studies are less useful than the community ones due to (1) lower reliability of retrospective than prospective data, and (2) other data limitations (fixed list of symptoms queried, little age detail in published results, highly-aggregated symptom groups). These comments should not dissuade readers from harvesting their worth, or looking at other studies of symptoms based on retrospective interviews, such as Brody and Kleban (1983) and others reviewed in Verbrugge and Ascione (1987: section "Symptoms Experienced by Adults").

12. This statement is for Detroit, where respondents were asked to name the condition causing their symptoms. Not known for Southfield.

13. Except Detroit, 65+: This anomaly may be partly due to narrowing sex differences at older ages, partly to unstable rates from the small samples of older men and women.

14. The sample sizes of the studies hamper numerical comparisons of men's vs. women's rates for particular symptoms.

15. The original scheme has prompted extensive discussion and critique. Survey researchers have revamped it along the lines stated in the text.

16. Traditional epidemiology is concerned with risk factors for *disease*; this new brand of epidemiology is interested in risk factors for *disability*, given disease presence.

17. In some discussions, gross mobility items (walking, getting outside) and urinary/bladder continence are included as ADLs. However, most contemporary researchers consider mobility a very different concept (we include it with physical disability), and view incontinence as a disease condition.

18. For some empirical insight into this, see Spector et al. (1987).

19. Normally, IADL-difficulty rates exceed ADL-difficulty rates, since the IADL activities are more complex and more readily impeded by disease. The wording used in the Supplement on Aging (Table 2.14) counts people who do not perform an IADL for reasons besides health as NA (not ascertained); for example, someone whose wife manages household money. For the IADL rates, they stay in the denominator but are not in the numerator. If asked "could you," some of them would have said "No, I really couldn't, due to my condition X," and IADL rates would rise accordingly. Thus, the IADL rates shown are extremely conservative and oddly *lower* than some ADL rates.

20. For questions aimed at persons under age 45, see *Vital and Health Statistics*, Series 10, No. 160, (DHHS Publ. No. [PHS] 86-1588).

21. Readers will note that difficulty and dependence are mixed in the data series on major activity. They are fundamentally different perspectives of disability and should be kept separate. Besides such theoretical considerations, putting them together inevitably causes discontinuities in a series of rates.

22. Readers will find the same patterns of sex differences among whites and blacks in *Vital and Health Statistics*, Series 3, No. 25,(DHHS Publ. No. [PHS] 87-1409), Table 14.

23. In contrast to the unusual situation in Table 14, here we see IADL rates exceed ADL rates—as they should.

24. A third question: Given the presence of limiting X, what is the chance of severe, rather than mild or moderate, limitation? We do not address this in this section due to absence of relevant data.

25. Readers may freely continue comparisons of Tables 8 and 16. The classification schemes used for condition titles are very similar, though not identical.

26. The 21 titles are a more condensed form of the classifications in Tables 8 and 16. The advantage is having *exactly* the same scheme for prevalence, limitation, and limiting potential figures. Readers should not try to make detailed comparisons of Tables 17 and 18 with Tables 8 and 15.

27. These studies vary in how they operationalize disability/nondisability. Typically, the rule is that people exit from nondisabled status when they become dependent in ADLs, become institutionalized, or die.

28. This statement pertains to people living at both to and t₁. If everyone surveyed at to is considered, whether alive or dead at t₁, then "disability incidence" rates look higher for men. But this is only because they are much more likely to die than women.

29. Most people living in institutions do, in fact, have trouble performing ADLs. See *Vital and Health Statistics*, Series 3, No. 25, (DHHS Publ. No. [PHS] 87-1409), Table 59; and Series 13, No. 43, (DHEW Publ. No. [PHS] 79-1794), Table 23.

30. How the four difficulty/dependency rates line up is not certain; the author welcomes information on this.

REFERENCES

Branch, L. G., & Jette, A. M. (1982). A prospective study of long-term care institutionalization among the aged. *American Journal of Public Health, 72,* 1373-1379.

Branch L. G., Katz, S., Kniepmann, K., & Papsidero, J. A. (1984). A prospective study of functional status among community elders. *American Journal of Public Health, 74,* 266-268.

Branch, L. G., & Meyers, A. R. (1987). Assessing physical function in the elderly. *Clinics in Geriatric Medicine, 3,* 29-51.

Brody, E. M., & Kleban, M. H. (1983). Day-to-day mental and physical health symptoms of older people: A report on health logs. *The Gerontologist, 28,* 75-85.

Chapman, S. H., LaPlante, M.P., & Wilensky, G .R. (1986). Life expectancy and health status of the aged. *Social Security Bulletin, 49*(10), 24-48.

Collins, J. G. (1986). Prevalence of selected chronic conditions, United States, 1979-81. *Vital and Health Statistics* (Series 10, No. 155. DHHS Publ. No. [PHS] 86-1583). Hyattsville, MD: National Center for Health Statistics.

Cornoni-Huntley, J. C., Foley, D. J., White, L. R., Suzman, R., Berkman, L. F., Evans, D. A., & Wallace, R. B. (1985). Epidemiology of disability in the oldest old: Methodologic issues and preliminary findings. *Milbank Memorial Fund Quarterly/ Health and Society, 63,* 350-376.

Crimmins, E. M. (1981). The changing patterns of American mortality decline, 1940-77, and its implications for the future. *Population and Development Review, 7,* 229-254.

Crimmins, E. M. (1984). Life expectancy and the older population. *Research on Aging, 6,* 490-514.

Crimmins, E. M., & Saito, Y. (1987). *Changes in life expectancy and disability free life expectancy in the U.S.: 1970-1980.* Paper presented at the Population Association of America meetings, 1988, Crimmins: Andrus Gerontology Center, University Park MC-0191, Los Angeles, CA.

Dawson, D., Hendershot, G., & Fulton, J. (1987). Aging in the eighties: Functional limitations of individuals age 65 years and over. *Advance Data,* No. 133. Hyattsville, MD: National Center of Health Statistics.

Faber, J. F., & Wade, A. H. (1983). Life Tables for the United States: 1900-2050. *Actuarial Study.* (No. 89. SSA Publ. No. 11-11536). Washington, DC: Social Security Administration.

Feldman, J. J. (1983). Work ability of the aged under conditions of improving mortality. *Milbank Memorial Fund Quarterly/Health and Society, 61*, 430-444.

Feller, B. A. (1983). Americans needing help to function at home. *Advance Data*, No. 92. Hyattsville, MD: National Center for Health Statistics.

Fingerhut, L. A. (1982). Changes in mortality among the elderly, United States, 1940-78. *Vital and Health Statistics.* (Series 3, No. 22. DHHS Publ. No. [PHS] 82-1406). And, Supplement to 1980. *Vital and Health Statistics.* (Series 3, No. 22a. DHHS Publ. No. [PHS] 84-1406a). 1984. Hyattsville, MD: National Center for Health Statistics.

Foley, D. J., Berkman, L. F., Branch, L. G., Farmer, M. E., & Wallace, R. B. (1986). Physical functioning. In J. Cornoni-Huntley, D. B. Brock, A. M. Ostfeld, J. O. Taylor, & R. B. Wallace (Eds.), *Established populations for epidemiologic studies of the elderly: Resource Data Book* (pp. 56-94). (NIH Publication No. 86-2443). Bethesda, MD: National Institute on Aging.

Gold, E. B. (Ed.). (1984). *The changing risk of disease in women: An epidemiologic approach.* Lexington, MA: D.C. Heath.

Guralnik, J. M. (1987). Capturing the full range of physical functioning in older populations. In *Proceedings of the 1987 Public Health Conference on Records and Statistics* (pp. 236-240). (DHHS Publ. No. [PHS] 88-1214). Hyattsville, MD: National Center for Health Statistics.

Haber, L. D. (1971). Disabling effects of chronic disease and impairment. *Journal of Chronic Diseases, 24*, 469-487.

Haber, L. D. (1973). Disabling effects of chronic disease and impairment - II. Functional capacity limitations. *Journal of Chronic Diseases, 26*, 127-151.

Haug, M. R., Ford, A. B., & Sheafor, M. (Eds.). (1985). *The physical and mental health of aged women.* New York: Springer.

Havlik, R. J., Liu, B. M., Kovar, M. G., Suzman, R., Feldman, J. J., Harris, T. & Van Nostrand, J. (1987). Health statistics on older persons, United States, 1986. *Vital and Health Statistics.* (Series 3, No. 25. DHHS Publ. No. [PHS] 87-1409). Hyattsville, MD: National Center for Health Statistics.

Haynes, S. G. & Feinleib, M. (Eds.). (1980). *Second conference on the epidemiology of aging.* (NIH Publ. No. 80-969). Bethesda, MD: National Institute on Aging.

Hazzard, W. R. (1984). The sex differential in longevity. In R. Andres, E. L. Bierman, & W. R. Hazzard (Eds.), *Principles of geriatric medicine* (pp. 72-81). New York: McGraw-Hill.

Hing, E. (1981). Characteristics of nursing home residents, health status, and care received: National nursing home survey, United States, May-December 1977. *Vital and Health Statistics.* (Series 13, No. 51. DHHS Publ. No. [PHS] 81-1712). Hyattsville, MD: National Center for Health Statistics.

Hing, E., & Cypress, B. K. (1981). Use of health services by women 65 years of age and over, United States. *Vital and Health Statistics.* (Series 13, No. 59. DHHS Publ. No. [PHS] 81-1720). Hyattsville, MD: National Center for Health Statistics.

Hing, E., Kovar, M. G., & Rice, D. P. (1983). Sex differences in health and use of medical care, United States, 1979. *Vital and Health Statistics.* (Series 3, No. 24. DHHS Publ. No. [PHS] 83-1408). Hyattsville, MD: National Center for Health Statistics.

Holden, C. (1987). Why do women live longer than men? *Science, 9 October*,158-160.

Jette, A. M., & Branch, L. G. (1981). The Framingham Disability Study: II. Physical disability among the aging. *American Journal of Public Health, 71*, 1211-1216.

Jette, A. M., & Branch, L. G. (1984). Musculoskeletal impairment among the non-institutionalized aged. *International Rehabilitation Medicine, 6*, 157-161.

Katz, S., & Akpom, C. A. (1976). A measure of primary sociobiological functions. *International Journal of Health Services, 6*, 493-507.

Katz, S., Branch, L. G., Branson, M. H., Papsidero, J. A., Back, J. C., & Greer, D. S. (1983). Active life expectancy. *New England Journal of Medicine, 309*, 1218-1224.

Klebba, A. J., Maurer, J. D., & Glass, E. J. (1973). Mortality trends: Age, color, and sex, United States, 1950-69. *Vital and Health Statistics*. (Series 20, No. 15. DHEW Publ. No. [HRA] 74-1852). Rockville, MD: National Center for Health Statistics.

LaLonde, M. (1975). *A new perspective on the health of Canadians*. Ottawa: Information Canada.

LaPlante, M. P. (1988). *Data on disability from the National Health Interview Survey, 1983-85*. Washington, DC: National Institute on Disability and Rehabilitation Research, U.S. Dept. of Education.

Liu, K., & Manton, K. G. (1987). Long-term care: Current estimates and projections. *Proceedings of the 1987 Public Health Conference on Records and Statistics* (pp. 102-104). (DHHS Publ. No. [PHS] 88-1214). Hyattsville, MD: National Center for Health Statistics.

Lopez, A. D., & Ruzicka, L. T. (Eds.). (1983). *Sex differentials in mortality: Trends, determinants, and consequences*. (Miscellaneous Series No. 4). Canberra, Australia: Department of Demography, Australian National University.

Macken, C. L. (1986). A profile of functionally impaired elderly persons living in the community. *Health Care Financing Review, 7*, 33-49.

Manton, K. G. (1988). *Sex differences in functional impairment in the U.S. elderly population: The interaction of specific diseases, functional impairments, and mortality*. Paper presented at the Population Association of America meetings, 1988, Center for Demographic Studies, Duke University, Durham, NC.

Manton, K. G., & Soldo, B. J. (1985). Dynamics of health changes in the oldest old: New perspectives and evidence. *Milbank Memorial Fund Quarterly/Health and Society, 63*, 206-285.

McMillen, M. M., & Rosenberg, H. M. (1983). Trends in United States mortality. *Proceedings of the American Statistical Association (Social Statistics Section)* pp. 88-92.

Mechanic, D. (1976). Sex, illness, illness behavior, and the use of health services. *Social Science and Medicine, 12B*, 207-214.

Metropolitan Life Insurance Co. (1987). New high for expectation of life. *Statistical Bulletin, 68(3)*, 8-14.

Metropolitan Life Insurance Co. (1988). Women's longevity advantage declines. *Statistical Bulletin, 69(1)*, 18-23.

Moss, A. J., & Parsons, V. L. (1986). Current estimates from the National Health Interview Survey, United States, 1985. *Vital and Health Statistics*. (Series 10, No. 160. DHHS Publ. No. [PHS] 86-1588). Hyattsville, MD: National Center for Health Statistics.

Nagi, S. Z. (1976). An epidemiology of disability among adults in the United States. *Milbank Memorial Fund Quarterly/Health and Society, 54*, 439-467.

Nathanson, C. A. (1977). Sex, illness, and medical care: A review of data, theory, and method. *Social Science and Medicine, 11*, 13-25.

Nathanson, C. A. (1984). Sex differences in mortality. In R. H. Turner & J. F. Short (Eds.), *Annual Review of Sociology*, (Vol. 10, pp. 191-213). Palo Alto, CA: Annual Reviews.

Nathanson, C. A., & Lorenz, G. (1982). Women and health: The social dimensions of biomedical data. J. Z. Giele (Ed.), *Women in the middle years* (pp. 37-87). New York: John Wiley.

Olshansky, S. J., & Ault, A. B. (1986). The fourth stage of the epidemiologic transition: The age of delayed degenerative diseases. *Milbank Memorial Fund Quarterly/Health and Society, 64*, 355-391.

Preston, S. H. (1976). *Older male mortality and cigarette smoking*. Westport, CT: Greenwood Press.

Proprietary Association, The. (1984). *Health care practices and perceptions. A consumer survey of self-medication*. Washington, DC: (Office of Public Affairs, The Proprietary Association, 1700 Pennsylvania Ave., N.W., Suite 700, ZIP 20006).

Retherford, R. D. (1975). *The changing sex differential in mortality*. Westport, CT: Greenwood Press.

Rice, D. P., & Feldman, J. J. (1983). Living longer in the United States: Demographic changes and health needs of the elderly. *Milbank Memorial Fund Quarterly/Health and Society, 61*, 362-396.

Rice, D. P., & LaPlante, M. P. (1988). Chronic illness, disability, and increasing longevity. In S. Sullivan & M. E. Lewin (Eds.), *Ethics and economics of long-term care*. Washington, DC: American Enterprise Institute.

Ries, P. W. (1983). Americans assess their health, United States, 1978. *Vital and Health Statistics*. (Series 10, No. 142. DHHS Publ. No. [PHS] 83-1570). Hyattsville, MD: National Center for Health Statistics.

Riley, M. W., & Bond, K. (1983). Beyond ageism: Postponing the onset of disability. In M. W. Riley, B. B. Hess, & K. Bond (Eds.), *Aging in society: Selected reviews of recent research* (pp. 243-252). Hillsdale, NJ: Lawrence Erlbaum.

Robine, J. M., Colvez, A., Bucquet, D., Hatton, F., Morel, B., & Lelaidier, S. (1986). L'esperance de vie sans incapacite en France en 1982. *Population, 6*, 1025-1042.

Rogers, A., Rogers, R. G., & Branch, L. G. (in press). A multistate analysis of active life expectancy. *Public Health Reports*.

Rosenwaike, I. (1985a). *The extreme aged in America*. Westport, CT: Greenwood Press.

Rosenwaike, I. (1985b). A demographic portrait of the oldest old. *Milbank Memorial Fund Quarterly/Health and Society, 63*, 187-205.

Rosenwaike, I., Yaffe, N. & Sagi, P. C. (1980). The recent decline in mortality of the extreme aged: An analysis of statistical data. *American Journal of Public Health, 70*, 1074-1080.

Schneider, D., Appleton, L., & McLemore, T. (1979). A reason for visit classification for ambulatory care. *Vital and Health Statistics*. (Series 2, No. 78. DHEW Publ. No. [PHS] 79-1352). Hyattsville, MD: National Center for Health Statistics.

Shanas, E. (1962). *The health of older people*. Cambridge, MA: Harvard University Press.

Shanas, E. (1968). Health and incapacity in later life. In E. Shanas, P. Townsend, D. Wedderburn, H. Friis, P. Milhoj, & J. Stehouwer (Eds.), *Old people in three industrial societies* (pp. 18-48). New York: Atherton Press.

Siegel, J. S. (1979). Prospective trends in the size and structure of the elderly population, impact of mortality trends, and some implications. *Current Population Reports* (Series P-23, No. 78). Washington, DC: U.S. Bureau of the Census.

Siegel, J. S., & Davidson, M. (1984). Demographic and socioeconomic aspects of aging in the United States. *Current Population Reports* (Series P-23, No. 138). Washington, DC: Bureau of the Census.

Soldo, B. J., & Manton, K. G. (1985). Health status and service needs of the oldest old: Current patterns and future trends. *Milbank Memorial Fund Quarterly/Health and Society, 63,* 286-319.

Spector, W. D., Katz, S., Murphy, J. B., & Fulton, J. P. (1987). The hierarchical relationship between activities of daily living and instrumental activities of daily living. *Journal of Chronic Diseases, 6,* 481-489.

Taeuber, C. M. (1983). America in transition: An aging society. *Current Population Reports* (Series P-23, No. 128). Washington, DC: U.S. Bureau of the Census.

U.S. Senate Special Committee on Aging. (1986). *Aging America, trends and projections* (1985-1986 Ed.). Washington, DC: U.S. Senate.

Verbrugge, L. M. (1976a). Sex differentials in morbidity and mortality in the United States. *Social Biology, 23,* 275-296.

Verbrugge, L. M. (1976b). Females and illness: Recent trends in sex differences in the United States. *Journal of Health and Social Behavior, 17,* 387-403.

Verbrugge, L. M. (1980). Recent trends in sex mortality differentials in the United States. *Women and Health, 5,* 17-37.

Verbrugge, L. M. (1982). Sex differentials in health. *Public Health Reports, 97,* 417-437.

Verbrugge, L. M. (1983). Women and men: Mortality and health of older people. In M. W. Riley, B. B. Hess, & K. Bond (Eds.), *Aging in society: Selected reviews of recent research* (pp. 139-174). Hillsdale, NJ: Lawrence Erlbaum.

Verbrugge, L. M. (1984a). A health profile of older women with comparisons to older men. *Research on Aging, 6,* 291-322.

Verbrugge, L. M. (1984b). Longer life but worsening health? Trends in health and mortality of middle-aged and older persons. *Milbank Memorial Fund Quarterly/Health and Society, 62,* 475-519.

Verbrugge, L. M. (1985a). An epidemiological profile of older women. In M. R. Haug, A. B. Ford, & M. Sheafor (Eds.), *The physical and mental health of aged women* (pp. 41-64). New York: Springer.

Verbrugge, L. M. (1985b). Gender and health: An update on hypotheses and evidence. *Journal of Health and Social Behavior, 26,* 156-182.

Verbrugge, L. M. (1987). From sneezes to adieux: Stages of health for American men and women. In R. A. Ward & S. S. Tobin (Eds.), *Health in aging: Sociological issues and policy directions* (pp. 17-57). New York: Springer.

Verbrugge, L. M. (1988). Unveiling higher morbidity for men: The story. In M. W. Riley (Ed.), *Social change and the life course.* Vol. 1: *Social change and human lives* (pp. 138-160). American Sociological Presidential Volume. Newbury Park, CA: Sage.

Verbrugge, L. M. (1989). Recent, present, and future health of American adults. In L. Breslow, J. E. Fielding, & L. B. Lave (Eds.), *Annual Review of Public Health* (Vol. 10). Palo Alto, CA: Annual Reviews.

Verbrugge, L. M. (in press). The twain meet: Empirical explanations of sex differences in health and mortality. *Journal of Health and Social Behavior.*

Verbrugge, L. M., & Ascione, F. J. (1987). Exploring the iceberg: Common symptoms and how people care for them. *Medical Care, 25,* 539-569.

Verbrugge, L. M., & Wingard, D. L. (1987). Sex differentials in health and mortality. *Women and Health, 12,* 103-145.

Waldron, I. (1976). Why do women live longer than men? *Social Science and Medicine, 10*, 349-362.

Waldron, I. (1982). An analysis of causes of sex differences in mortality and morbidity. In W. R. Gove & G. R. Carpenter (Eds.), *The fundamental connection between nature and nurture.* Lexington, MA: D.C. Heath.

Waldron, I. (1983a). Sex differences in human mortality: The role of genetic factors. *Social Science and Medicine, 17*, 321-333.

Waldron, I. (1983b). Sex differences in illness incidence, prognosis, and mortality: Issues and evidence. *Social Science and Medicine, 17*, 1107-1123.

Waldron, I. (1986a). What do we know about causes of sex differences in mortality? A review of the literature. *Population Bulletin of the United Nations, 18*, 59-76.

Waldron, I. (1986b). The contribution of smoking to sex differences in mortality. *Public Health Reports, 101*, 163-173.

Ward, R. A., & Tobin, S. S. (Eds.). (1987). *Health in aging: Sociological issues and policy directions.* New York: Springer.

Wilkins, R., & Adams, O. B. (1983a). Health expectancy in Canada, late 1970's: Demographic, regional, and social dimensions. *American Journal of Public Health, 73*, 1073-1080.

Wilkins, B., & Adams, O. B. (1983b). *Healthfulness of life.* Montreal: The Institute for Research and Public Policy.

Wingard, D. L. (1982). The sex differential in mortality rates. *American Journal of Epidemiology, 115*, 205-216.

Wingard, D. L. (1984). The sex differential in morbidity, mortality, and lifestyle. L. Breslow, J. E. Fielding, & L. B. Lave (Eds.), *Annual review of public health.* (Vol. 5, pp. 433-458). Palo Alto, CA: Annual Reviews.

Wingard, D. L., Suarez, L., & Barrett-Connor, E. (1983). The sex differential in mortality from all causes and ischemic heart disease. *American Journal of Epidemiology, 117*, 165-172

World Health Organization. (1980). *International classification of impairments, disabilities, and handicaps.* Geneva.

World Health Organization. (1984). The uses of epidemiology in the study of the elderly. *Technical Report Series*, No. 706. Geneva.

Yelin, E. H. (in press). The social context of the work disability problem. *Milbank Memorial Fund Quarterly/Health and Society.*

Zopf, P. E., Jr. (1986). *America's older population.* Houston, TX: Cap and Gown Press.

CHAPTER 3

Class, Aging, and Health

CHARLES F. LONGINO, Jr.
GEORGE J. WARHEIT
JULIE ANN GREEN

INTRODUCTION

The essential reason for this chapter is to determine if, (and if so) to what degree, social class is associated with health among the elderly in the United States. Because gender, race, and ethnicity are covered in other chapters, this treatment of social class does not attempt to partial out the variance from, or consider interaction with, those other explanatory variables.

It has been found repeatedly in recent years, and documented in other chapters, that many predictors of health and mortality do not predict as well in old age. In fact, some of these associations may even reverse themselves in advanced old age as in the case of race. This is probably the outcome of some kind of selective survival. Where there is not a strong association between class and health in old age, it might be explained in terms of such selection factors. In the pages that follow, after discussing the concepts and the data that will be used to explore their relationships, social class measures will be tabulated with basic demographic variables to profile the social class categories. Then, general mortality and major causes of death by social class will be discussed. The literature on these topics is very thin. Disease preva-

AUTHORS, NOTE: This chapter would not have been written without the long hours and hard work of Dawn Leeds, Frances Cutler, Bill LeBlanc, and Jennifer Schmitt. The analysis was supported in part by a grant from the AARP Andrus Foundation.

asses will be explored, both for major diseases,
/ar disease, stroke, and cancer, and for chronic
ons that are less serious. Finally, functional health
ratings will be examined in the social class catego-
)n will be given to medical care and community
socioeconomic groupings in the context of functional
in overall assessment will be made concerning the
relationship ween social class and health among the elderly, and
some topics for additional research will be suggested.

CONCEPTUAL CONSIDERATIONS

A reasoned consideration of aging and health must begin by exploring the concepts. Age affects health in at least three ways (Palmore,
1978). The most obvious effect comes from biological aging, the
change in an organism over time after growth has ended. Senescence is
one effect of age on health. At its optimum, senescence is the gradual
decline of organs, functions, and capacities in a trajectory determined
only by genetics. We do not live under optimum health conditions,
however. Therefore, the other two effects of age on health come into play.

The second effect comes from the shared life experience of one's
age peers in society. In the late 1980s, persons in their late sixties in the
United States, for example, can bill the federal government for many
of their doctor and hospital bills. Persons in their late sixties before
1965 did not have medicare, and a century ago they did not experience
hospital-based medical care and third-party payments at all (Palmore,
1986).

The cohort effect of age on health is apparent when one examines
the health of persons in a broad age range, for example, among people
over age 55. Part of the health differences between those in their late
fifties and those in their early eighties is due to senescence. Some of it,
however, has to do with other differences between persons in the
younger and older categories. The understanding of health that was
available to the younger group during its young and middle adult years
was not available to the older group at the same age. To the extent that
health is influenced by diet and exercise, for example, the younger
group may have a healthier old age than the older group when it reaches
those advanced years. Health conditions and health practices have
improved over time, increasing, as a result, the effect of senescent

aging on health by reducing the insult of environmental factors on health. For this reason alone there is a cohort difference in health among the elderly (Riley, 1987).

The third effect of age on health has to do with the unevenness of the environment. A discussion of cohort effects always seems to assume a cultural uniformity and uniform access to health care. Exposure, willingness, acceptability, and opportunity are not evenly distributed either.

Many thousands of Americans will never reach old age because of their exposure to AIDS, a disease that was unknown a generation ago and for which there may be a cure a generation hence. If there is a cohort effect on health from this disease it is because persons in their young adult years are more readily exposed to it. Some are more or less likely to be exposed at any age, however, depending on their sexual behavior, which in turn is influenced by their sexual preferences, religious beliefs, and opportunities. Beyond senescence and cohort, age affects health differently depending on one's "life chances." There are different cohort effects on the health of promiscuous gay men and monogamous heterosexual women. Draft-age men in the mid-1960s had a different exposure to the negative health effects of war than did women of the same age. These differences in life chances alter the way in which the environment impacts health because they channel people differently into health relevant environments. What is often called a "period effect" in gerontology is rooted in the notion of life chances as it crosscuts the cohort dimension.

This volume looks at age effects on the health of older people. But more importantly, it takes into account, one by one, the major factors that affect the health-relevant environmental opportunities of people. Social class is certainly one of these.

The concept of social inequality will breathe life into the term "social class" in this discussion. Social class does not refer to caste or fixed social strata. It only refers to the fact that classes or categories will be developed to allow us to use social inequality as a meaningful variable. Notions of upper, middle, and lower class, as though they are identifiable, mutually exclusive, and meaningful social categories, are not useful distinctions here. The underlying concept is life chances, those resources whose presence enhances one's opportunities for a healthy old age and whose limitation or absence hinders it.

It is important to understand that health, class, and age change over time, a point to which we will return again later. It is easy to see that age changes on a personal level. It is more critical, however, to understand that it also changes on a societal level. If people in their sixties today are healthier, better educated, and economically more secure than they were a generation or two ago, then they will seem younger than people of the same age did then. In this sense, perhaps, the aging process is slowing down.

Health is changing, too. Health practices and health care are changing. In addition, the workplace and the home are healthier environments than they once were. We are simply more health conscious, conscious of those factors that affect our health, and it is more acceptable than in past decades to act on that knowledge to keep ourselves healthy. In this sense, health changes. We live in healthier times.

Finally, social class also changes. It changes on a personal level as individuals advance their own education and their economic standing to levels that are ever higher. On a societal level, also, the average number of years of education is increasing, and the entry-level requirements for jobs are also increasing. The social value of education has inflated so that essentially the same social ranking may require more education with each passing generation. Status inflation not withstanding, there is still a net increase in life chances due to better education, especially as it impacts upon health, with each passing generation. And in that sense, social class changes over time, just as age and health do.

Age, class, and health interact with one another as a social policy issue (Soldo & Manton, 1985). The American people have come to expect to be healthy—as a right. They may choose unhealthy practices or conditions, but health *care* is something that workers expect employers and the government to pay for. They expect the government to protect their workplace from danger, their food from contamination, and their environment from toxins—as a right. In old age, they expect the burden of the employer to shift to the government. It is their right as citizens, regardless of age or social class. The health care of the poor should be subsidized if necessary beyond that of others. It is their right. The implication for life chances of this drift toward greater health protection and care access is obvious (Barsky, 1988).

It is population aging, not just personal aging, that threatens to collide with expanding health rights (Longino & Soldo, 1987). Some fear that the growth of the very old population in this country could become too expensive a burden for the government to bear. If this eventually happens, there would be a health policy crisis of the first magnitude.

There is a public-private partnership implied in American health care policy; even with Medicare and Medicaid, the public sector pays the private sector to render medical services. The public sector has, in varying degrees, tended to make it possible for citizens to buy their health care on the open market. Medicare and Medicaid function as insurers of the health care of the elderly, as employers do for most adults before retirement. Underlying most of the issues associated with accommodating a rapidly aging population are concerns for equity. If the state views the elderly as a totally dependent population that it somehow has to "take care of," then a rapidly aging national population would first bring on a dull trauma, followed by a frenzied total panic. Fortunately, only a small part of this population, even of the oldest old, is totally dependent on public support. However, an even smaller part is completely independent of such help when Social Security is factored into the discussion. It is the *relative* proportion of the care burden that is shifted from private to public shoulders and back again that will frame the continuing public dialogue about equity (Soldo & Longino, 1988).

DATA

The National Health Interview Survey has been carried out by the National Center for Health Statistics (NCHS) for over 30 years. It is a large, continuing survey of the civilian non-institutionalized population in the United States. In 1984, a special supplement, the Supplement on Aging, was added to the national survey. This 30-minute interview following the general interview was designed to obtain special information about 16,148 people at age 55 and over who were living in the 42,000 households included in the national survey. This supplement produced an extensive file of data about the health of the older noninstitutionalized population and their chronic conditions and impairments. These are the data that were used to explore the relationship between social class and health among the elderly in the United States.

Creating a variable to measure socioeconomic status was a challenge. There were no data on the former occupations of the retired respondents in the supplement on aging. There were some elemental questions on education and income, however. They had to do. Percentile scores were derived for the education and the household income distributions separately. These percentile scores were added together and then repercentiled to produce four categories of socioeconomic status. This procedure resulted in a socioeconomic status score being assigned to every respondent in the study. The quartiles became the primary independent variable of the analysis.

We were fortunate to have a measure of poverty status already provided for each individual in the survey by the National Center for Health Statistics. Poverty status is the second major organizing variable for the analysis, which is broken into two categories, those above and those below the poverty threshold.

It is only fair to add a note at this point concerning the omission of occupational status as one of the defining variables of socioeconomic status. Occupational status is considered by many students of social inequality to be perhaps the major contributor to this concept. While income and education undergo a certain amount of inflation over time, as noted above, occupational rankings stay relatively stable in relationship to one another. It is obviously a weaker measure when occupational prestige ranking is left out. The data that were used in this analysis, however, did not provide former occupation for those who were retired. It makes no sense to rank the occupations of those younger subjects who were still employed and to set at zero the ranking of those who were retired, or who never worked outside their home. The choice was made, therefore, to do without occupation in the measure of socioeconomic status.

BASIC DEMOGRAPHIC OVERVIEW

There are two reasons for examining the association between social class measures and basic demographic variables. The purpose of this examination is twofold. First, it will allow us to assess the construct validity of the social class measures by comparing them (socioeconomic status and poverty status) with one another as they relate to the demographic variables.

There is a second reason for examining the demographic correlates of social class. When a bivariate association between health and social class is found, the reader's tendency is to reach for explanations beyond the class measures themselves, and to argue that social class is confounded by other explanatory variables, such as gender, age, race, and ethnicity. Each of the chapters in this book focuses on one explanatory variable. Therefore, any discussion of the interaction between gender, race, ethnicity, and social class as they affect the health of older people runs the risk of generating border disputes. This

TABLE 3.1 Demographic Characteristics by Social Class

| | Socioeconomic Quartiles | | | | Poverty Level | |
	Lowest	Second	Third	Highest	Below	Above
Age						
55-64 Yrs.	12.6	25.6	47.0	58.9	22.0	30.6
65-74 Yrs.	43.5	52.7	41.7	31.9	40.4	44.9
75+ Yrs.	43.9	21.8	11.3	9.2	37.7	24.5
Gender						
Male	37.2	48.5	45.5	54.1	29.2	44.8
Female	62.8	51.5	54.5	46.0	70.8	55.2
Marital Status						
Married	39.1	73.5	79.6	88.7	30.2	65.8
Widowed	44.6	19.6	14.2	9.7	48.9	24.3
Divorced	6.2	2.7	2.4	1.1	8.9	4.2
Separated	3.0	0.6	0.7	0.0	3.7	1.0
Never Married	5.9	2.6	2.6	0.5	6.8	4.0
Employment						
Not Employed	90.8	79.6	63.8	44.9	87.9	72.5
Private Co.	5.3	13.3	22.2	32.4	7.2	16.3
Government*	1.1	2.6	5.6	8.1	1.2	4.2
Inc. Business	0.1	0.2	1.6	7.6	0.1	1.4
Self-Employed	2.1	3.8	5.7	6.0	3.0	4.7
Income Sources						
for the Retired						
Social Security	74.5	54.1	50.5	40.4	78.0	54.4
S.S. and Other	21.8	37.4	37.0	38.3	17.3	37.4
Other In. Only	3.5	8.5	12.5	21.3	4.4	8.0

*Includes federal, state, and local governments.

limitation makes it important to take a look at the demographic correlates of social class because their interaction may indeed affect health.

Table 3.1 displays the age, gender, marital status, employment, and income source differentials of persons in each of the socioeconomic quartiles and poverty levels. It is clear at a glance that the two social class measures have face validity.

There is a large age range among the respondents to the health survey. Age is not strongly related to poverty status; there is not a strong difference in the age distribution of those above and below the poverty level.

The variation is more obvious in the display of socioeconomic quartiles. Forty-four percent of the persons in the lowest SES quartile are 75 years of age or older. Only 9 percent of the highest quartile are in the oldest age category. Conversely, the youngest subjects, age 55-64, are under-represented in the lowest quartile (13 percent), and a majority of the persons in the highest quartile are in the youngest age category.

There are several reasons that the oldest are the poorest and the youngest are the wealthiest. There is a birth cohort factor at work here. Social Security retirement benefits and pensions covered fewer persons in the older age group than is true of recent retirees. Not only the coverage but the benefits to the older benefactors are less, on the whole, than they are to benefactors who are younger.

Another factor is the impact of retirement on income. Over 90 percent of the persons in the lowest quartile are no longer employed. In contrast, only 45 percent of the persons in the highest quartile are no longer employed. The income from salary and wages, or self-employment, is usually larger than are retirement benefits at the time when a person retires. Because the likelihood of retirement increases with age, and retirement usually brings a decline in income, advancing age (in the sixties) then is statistically related to changing socioeconomic status, independently from cohort explanations.

Because age is inversely related to income in the retirement years, one would expect to find social class measures inversely related to those diseases, such as cancer, whose prevalence increases with old age. In such cases it may not be social class that is related to cancer but age, which is associated with social class through income.

Gender is a second demographic variable shown in Table 3.1 that is associated with social class. Over 70 percent of the poor, as measured by poverty level, are women as compared to only 55 percent of those who are not poor. The quartile measure, with its greater number of categories, shows a stronger association with gender. Nearly two-thirds of those in the lowest socioeconomic quartile are women, and the majority of those in the highest quartile are men. The socioeconomic statuses of men and women are similar in the second and third quartiles. It is, thus, the richest quartile where the gender difference is pronounced.

These differences, of course, call to mind the feminization of poverty in old age (Minkler & Stone, 1985). A study of the population characteristics of very old men and women (Longino, 1987a), using

1980 census data, found that a higher proportion of men than women received income from nearly every source identified in the census: salaries and wages, self-employment, social security, assets, and other income, including pensions. The only exception was income from public assistance and Supplemental Social Security Income (SSI). Further, this study pointed out that when men and women who received income from each source were compared, the men had higher average incomes than the women, even from public assistance. The result of these comparisons is that when men and women over age 85 were compared, the men had a 20 percent higher personal income from all sources than did women. It is important to remember that gender is associated with age when considering the effect of social class on health among the elderly. The older the age category, the greater will be the proportion of women. For example, only 31 percent of the population over age 85 are men. One of the reasons that socioeconomic status is negatively associated with age, as seen in Table 3.1, is that women have lower incomes on the whole than men do, and that women outlive men at higher rates with advancing age.

Women at the same ages are less healthy than men; morbidity levels are higher among women than among men. Furthermore, men tend to die at younger ages than women, as noted above; mortality levels are higher among men. Finally, women tend to have lower socioeconomic status than men. One could argue that as a result of the interaction of these three factors, measures of functional dependency and disability should be indirectly associated with social class. The issue of confounding explanatory variables again arises.

Marital status is the third demographic variable shown in Table 3.1. Being married seems to be strongly associated with socioeconomic status and negatively associated with poverty. Nearly two-thirds of the persons who live in households with incomes above the poverty level are married. Roughly twice the proportion of each of the other marital statuses (widowed, separated, divorced, and never married) are found in the below poverty column.

The marital status differentials among the quartiles of socioeconomic status add more detail to the bivariate association. Nearly nine out of ten persons in the highest quartile of socioeconomic status are married. But with descending quartiles, the proportion does not drop sharply until the poorest quartile is reached. Fewer than two-fifths of the individuals in this category are married. The same pattern is seen in reverse for the other marital statuses. The widowed, divorced, separated, and never married are proportionately concentrated in the poorest quartile of socioeconomic status.

Marital status does not stand alone as an explanatory variable associated with social class. It is nested in a set of variables including age and gender. With each advancing age category, one will find fewer married persons and more widows. Since mortality rates are higher for men, this means that more women are widowed. The relationship is the strongest among the very old (Longino, 1988). Longino (1987a) found that in the advanced years (over age 85) nearly half of the men were married but fewer than a tenth of the women were married. This is an extremely large disparity, but the reasons for it are relatively straightforward. The remarriage rate of men after widowhood far exceeds that of women. Women are apt to become widowed partly because husbands tend to be older than wives. Marital status may be associated with social class indirectly through the age and gender connection. Its potential effect upon the relationship between social class and health is not as clear as that of age and gender.

Not surprisingly, those who are employed have a social class advantage through income. Over half of the persons in the highest socioeconomic quartile are employed. The employment factor may in good part account for the elevated levels of social class among persons in the youngest age category and among men.

Finally, it should be noted that those persons who rely on Social Security as their only source of income in old age are more likely to be found among the poor than those who rely on a combination of income sources or on sources other than Social Security. Persons who indicated no source of income were left out of this tabulation.

This chapter asks whether social class affects health among the elderly. In the introduction to this chapter the effects of age on health were discussed, and social class was introduced as a form of social inequality involving those resources whose presence enhances one's opportunities for a healthy old age and whose limitation or absence hinders it. Conceiving social class so broadly enhances the limitations of its measurement, especially in the context of secondary data analysis, relying on such concepts as poverty, education, and income.

A profile emerges from the demographic overview. The most advantaged segments of the study population are employed, married men in their late fifties and early sixties. The most disadvantaged segments are widowed women over age 75 relying only on Social Security for their income.

The two measures of social class seem to work well together. They describe the same patterns. However, the socioeconomic quartiles spread out the variation more, making it the more useful of the two measures.

It is very evident in the presentation of the demographic overview that the "resources whose presence enhance one's opportunities for a healthy old age and whose limitation or absence hinder it" are not discrete and independent. There are predisposing factors to social class just as there are to health. Widowed women over age 55 could be a surrogate measure of social class disadvantage just as married men in the same general age group could be a surrogate measure of social class advantage. Ethnicity and race could also be added to the list of associated demographic characteristics. When the simple bivariate association between social class and health is described, therefore, the simplicity of the relationship is more apparent than real. The possibility of confounds must always be kept in mind as the social class and health relationship is probed in the pages that follow.

Finally, it must also be remembered that the relationships between explanatory variables are not only complex but are also dynamic. The impact of age on health changes over time as does the impact of gender on social status. If the gap in income and education declines between the genders, the age categories, and the marital statuses, then the explanatory matrix will shift, reducing the complexity of the model and increasing the independence of social class as an explanatory factor. The cohort trends that are now evident seem to point in this direction. As the baby boom pushes into the older age categories, there is certain to be a decrease in the feminization of poverty in old age because education and income gaps will decline due to increased participation of women in today's labor force. Because the relationship between social class and health is both complex and dynamic, its continued study will be able to note and mark these changes and, in the process, to chart the changing matrix of social inequality in our society.

So what are we to conclude from this demographic overview? First, the composite picture of the socioeconomically advantaged and disadvantaged parts of the older population did emerge from the cross-tabulations. Second, the construct validity of the measures of socioeconomic status was assessed and their relative advantage discussed. Third, a strong warning about confounding explanatory variables was given before introducing health variables.

GENERAL MORTALITY AND LIFE EXPECTANCY

In 1980 the Department of Health and Social Security in Great Britain published a report on the inequalities in health. The Black Report, as it was called, dealt primarily with social class differences in health and suggested that class differences in health were not declining in Great Britain. Recently, Wilkinson (1986a) joined with other British epidemiologists to examine the veracity of the Black Report. One of the studies looked at the effect of government pensions on the mortality rates of the elderly (Wilkinson, 1986b). Noting that retired persons in England usually have other sources of income besides their state pensions, it was assumed that fluctuations in the real value of pensions will produce fluctuations in total incomes that may be associated with mortality rates. The results were surprising, however. There were no significant correlations between death rates for the elderly and personal disposable income, per capita. After introducing several other controls, it was concluded that there must be diminishing health returns with increases in income. That is, pensions, in combination with other sources of income, provide an income floor that is high enough to diminish the effect of social class on mortality among older people in England. A comparison of English data with those in other Western countries and Japan seemed to support this conclusion.

Fox, Goldblatt, and Jones (1986) add a cautionary note from their research on social class mortality differentials. They warn that a drift downward on the economic scale may occur during periods of ill health. When social class is based on the occupation before retirement a decade or more before death, then occupationally based social class measures are not good predictors of mortality rates.

Finally, Marmot (1986) used British civil service grades as the measure of social class and examined the mortality rates of men who were approaching retirement (age 60-64). He found that social class, thus measured, was inversely related to general mortality rate.

To summarize, Wilkinson found that the public and private sectors contributed pension and non-pension income to the retired in such a way that mortality rates were not strongly associated with social class in old age, and that the same generalization could probably be made of the older population in Western countries. Marmot found an occupational class difference in mortality rates for older working men, but this finding does not contradict those of Wilkinson. Finally, Fox et al. warn that measures of social class based on the former occupations of older men are not very useful in predicting their mortality rates.

Studies of the impact of social class upon mortality rates among the elderly in the United States have had reinforcing if not identical results. It is possible, of course, that differences in the income maintenance system of retirees in England and the United States would hinder the generalizability of the British studies to the United States. Nonetheless, Branch and Jette (1984) found that personal health practices (smoking, alcohol consumption, amount of sleep, physical activity) do predict mortality among adults, but this effect is severely diminished among persons in their seventies and eighties. This, of course, would have the effect of reducing class differences in mortality in old age as well. Verbrugge (1987, 1984) also points out that fatal diseases make their appearance in middle age and progress from then on, one result being that mortality rates are remarkably stable across age groups. Observing all ages, of course, there is a well-documented decline in estimated survival probabilities with less adequate family income (Berkman and Breslow, 1983; Kaplan, Haan, Syme, Minkler, & Winkleby, 1987).

Selective survival is one way of explaining the lack of evidence that there is a social class effect on mortality in old age (Markides and Machalek, 1984). There may be higher rates of selective survival in disadvantaged, high mortality populations that result in a greater proportion of healthy, very old people.

MAJOR CAUSES OF DEATH

Causes of death are frequently tabulated by demographic variables such as age, gender and race (Longino, 1987b). They are rarely tabulated by socioeconomic variables, however. One older study, however, throws some light on this subject. Kitagawa and Hauser (1968) found that disease-specific mortality rates for persons who died past the age of 65 do differ in some cases by education. Death by cancer was more prevalent among those with more education. The reason for this finding seems to be that persons with more education tend to live longer due to social class factors and cancer is a more frequent cause of death among long-lived populations.

The Longitudinal Study of Aging (1986), conducted by the National Center for Health Statistics, links the individual records of study respondents to those in the national death registry so that causes of death will be available on the records of respondents after their death. This innovation will make it possible for researchers to make cause of death a dependent variable in studies using this data set in the future. At the time of this writing, however, the mortality data are not yet available.

Speculation about the impact of social class on cause of death, of course, is possible. Poverty and its associated life-style factors would predict high rates of homicide and accidental deaths for men, but these causes of death tend to be concentrated at much younger ages than those of interest to gerontologists. Causes of death that are sensitive to nutritional factors should be higher among the poor and less well-educated. However, these causes of death may take their toll, also, at younger ages than would be studied in a book such as this. The survivors may be the tough ones, and the causes of their deaths may not vary much from those of higher social classes (Markides & Machalek, 1984).

PREVALENCE OF MAJOR DISEASES

Why should there be social class differences in the prevalence of major diseases, such as heart disease, stroke, and cancer? It was once believed that coronary heart disease was a disease of the rich due to the fact that the upper classes could afford to eat more red meat. As the standard of living has risen in the country so has the prevalence of heart disease (Susser & Watson, 1971). Disease prevalence among the poor was greater for epidemics and infectious diseases and pneumonia (Kitagawa, 1969).

The only study that specifically examined disease prevalence of the older population with an explicit social class focus was published by Guralnick (1967) in which she analyzed the 1961-1963 national health interview survey data. She compared the morbidity ratios (standardized by age, gender, and farm-nonfarm residence) of persons over age 65 with incomes below and above $3,000 in 1960. It was a straightforward income comparison. She found that the morbidity ratios of older persons with higher incomes were below the national average for heart conditions, and those with lower incomes were above the national average. Similar findings were noted when a series of chronic condi-

TABLE 3.2 Prevalence of Major Diseases by Social Class

| *Per 100* | *Socioeconomic Quartiles* | | | | *Poverty Level* | |
Population	*Lowest*	*Second*	*Third*	*Highest*	*Below*	*Above*
Coronary Heart Disease	4.4	4.6	3.9	3.8	4.4	4.5
Cerebrovascular Disease	7.8	5.9	2.9	1.6	8.1	5.0
Cancer	8.9	9.1	10.1	15.1	8.6	10.8

tions and impairments were observed. Reliance on a single indicator may be a problem in Guralnick's study, but at least ground was broken.

The prevalence of three major diseases is shown in Table 3.2: coronary heart disease, cerebrovascular disease (stroke), and cancer. Contrary to expectations, there is essentially no difference in the prevalence of coronary heart disease between persons in households with incomes above or below poverty. Even the socioeconomic quartiles are not sensitive to differences in the prevalence of coronary heart disease. If this is a disease of the rich, it is not evident in Table 3.2. Stroke, on the other hand, is strongly and inversely related to social class. Eight percent of those in the below-poverty category had experienced a stroke in the past year, as compared with five percent of those in the above-poverty category. The socioeconomic quartiles display a gradient running from fewer than 8 percent for the poorest quartile to fewer than two percent for the richest quartile.

Kitagawa and Hauser (1968) found that mortality from cancer was higher among the better educated segment of the population. The prevalence of cancer, as shown in Table 3.2, is higher for those in the higher education-income quartiles, as well. Kaplan et al. (1987) noted that the chance of survival from cancer decreases the lower the socioeconomic level for the United States population in general, so here again there may be an actual crossover effect of social class and health in the older age group.

There does seem to be a small social class effect on the prevalence of major diseases in the older population, at least to the extent that it can be demonstrated in a bivariate analysis. Stronger effects are observed in less life-threatening diseases and conditions.

TABLE 3.3 Chronic Conditions Among Adults Age 17+ According to Type of Condition and Family Income

Chronic Condition and Year (per 1,000 Population)	*Family Income*			
	Less Than $5,000	*$5,000-$9,999*	*$10,000-$14,999*	*$15,000 & More*
Arthritis, 1969	411.7	353.3	310.9	300.8
Asthma, 1970	41.4	32.6	—	—
Bronchitis, 1970	45.4	37.2	27.4	40.7
Diabetes, 1973	82.0	76.1	81.1	62.7
Heart Conditions, 1972	219.0	190.0	158.9	174.8
Hypertensive Disease*, 1972	216.1	179.5	192.6	161.4

SOURCE: Division of Health Interview Statistics, National Center for Health Statistics. Selected reports from the Health Interview Survey, Vital and Health Statistics, Series 10, and unpublished data from the Health Interview Survey.
*Without heart involvement.
NOTE: Data based on household interview of samples of the civilian noninstitutionalized population.

OTHER LESS SERIOUS CHRONIC DISEASES AND CONDITIONS

Kart (1985) collected into one table (Table 3.3) the prevalence rate, per thousand population, of persons age 17 and above in the United States, by four categories of family income. It is evident from the table that many chronic diseases are associated with social class, as measured by income. Except for chronic bronchitis, all of the relationships run in the same direction. Those who had lower family incomes had higher prevalence rates than those who had higher family incomes. This was the case with arthritis, asthma, diabetes, heart conditions, hypertension, back and spine impairments, and vision impairments. The negative effect of social class on the prevalence of chronic diseases and conditions is evident.

A similar set of diseases and conditions are seen in Table 3.4, using data from the 1984 Supplement on Aging of the National Health Interview Survey. Again, the prevalence rates (per hundred) tend to be higher in the lower socioeconomic quartiles and among those with household incomes below the poverty level.

Coronary heart disease was not associated with either measure of social class, but heart conditions were. They are the most prevalent among the sample respondents in the lower socioeconomic quartiles.

TABLE 3.4 Chronic Diseases and Conditions by Social Class

Per 100 Population	Socioeconomic Quartiles				Poverty Level	
	Lowest	*Second*	*Third*	*Highest*	*Below*	*Above*
Heart Conditions	17.6	18.7	13.0	11.3	19.0	17.0
Hypertension	49.6	42.3	38.3	26.5	51.3	40.3
Atherosclerosis	12.0	8.4	6.4	6.0	11.5	9.3
Diabetes	13.7	8.0	7.1	8.1	12.8	8.8
Varicose Veins	11.2	9.5	9.5	4.9	11.6	10.2
Arthritis	60.7	50.7	43.4	35.7	60.9	47.2
Osteoporosis	2.3	2.2	3.7	2.2	2.4	3.1

Atherosclerosis is negatively associated with social class as well. Hypertension and diabetes, two chronic diseases that are frequently found among the elderly, are also negatively associated with socioeconomic status. Even varicose veins and arthritis are more prevalent among the poor than among those with higher incomes. Of the diseases and conditions listed in Table 3.4, only osteoporosis showed no association with social class.

Perhaps it should not be surprising that national adult patterns should also hold for the elderly. Chronic diseases or conditions are not disabling, taken alone, but when they accumulate with increasing age, they can become very limiting in their impact on the life-style and life space of the aging adult. The increased prevalence among the survey respondents who fall into the lower quartiles also implies that these are the persons who may suffer from multiple chronic conditions.

Impairments to one's senses, especially blindness and deafness, may also burden some older persons as they age, limiting or altering their normal activities as a result. Table 3.5 shows the distribution of visual and hearing impairments among the socioeconomic quartiles and the poverty levels. Glaucoma and color blindness are as prevalent among the upper as the lower socioeconomic quartiles and among those with incomes above as those with incomes below the poverty level. Blindness and deafness, however, are negatively associated with social class. Here again, the quartile measure is more sensitive to deafness differentials than the poverty measure. Difficulties in seeing or hearing are also negatively associated with the social class measures, whether the degree of difficulty is large or small. Finally, cataracts, the most common sight impairment among the elderly, beyond near-sightedness, is

TABLE 3.5 Sensory Impairments by Social Class

| | Socioeconomic Quartiles | | | | Poverty Level | |
	Lowest	Second	Third	Highest	Below	Above
Visual Impairments (per 100)						
Blindness*	5.9	2.7	1.9	2.2	5.8	3.4
Some Difficulty	32.1	20.2	13.9	12.0	32.4	20.8
Much Difficulty	9.9	2.6	0.8	1.6	9.0	3.2
Cataract	20.2	12.5	8.9	10.8	18.7	13.3
Glaucoma	4.1	3.2	2.3	3.8	3.9	3.4
Color Blindness	2.1	2.8	1.4	2.7	2.2	2.2
Hearing Impairments (per 100)						
Deafness**	11.8	10.7	7.0	4.3	10.6	10.3
Some Difficulty	33.6	33.1	24.3	20.5	31.3	29.1
Much Difficulty	8.6	3.8	1.6	1.1	7.6	3.7

*In one or both eyes.
**In one or both ears.

far more prevalent among the economically disadvantaged. Impairments, like chronic conditions and diseases, can be multiplicative, giving the elderly person more than one problem with which to cope.

It is important to ask at this point whether the greater prevalence of chronic diseases and conditions and impairments is reflected in the use of health care services. Do those with higher or lower status use more services? Because office visits are not paid by medicare, perhaps there should be a positive association between the use of health care services and social class measures. Table 3.6 reveals that there is essentially no association at all between time of last doctor visit and the measures of social class. About four-fifths of all the persons in each of the quartiles have visited a physician during the past year. Nor is there any appreciable SES difference in rates of use of visiting nurses and health aides among the elderly who were surveyed by the National Center for Health Statistics. The prevalence was very low in all quartiles.

It is somewhat surprising that the prevalence rates of so many conditions and impairments would be higher in the lower SES categories, and yet no differences are seen in the pattern of health care use. The impact of medicare and medicaid on health care use may explain the absence of a social class effect.

TABLE 3.6 Use of Health Care Services by Social Class

| | Socioeconomic Quartiles | | | | Poverty Level | |
	Lowest	Second	Third	Highest	Below	Above
Time of Last Doctor Visit (%)						
Never	0.1	0.0	0.0	0.0	0.1	0.1
Less Than 1 Yr.	81.3	80.3	81.2	78.9	79.5	81.2
Between 1-2 Yrs.	5.9	5.7	5.8	9.7	5.9	6.3
Between 2-5 Yrs.	7.5	8.7	8.0	6.5	8.3	7.8
5 Yrs. or More	4.7	5.1	4.6	3.8	5.2	4.2
Other Services (%)						
Visiting Nurse	3.3	1.6	1.3	1.7	3.8	2.0
Health Aide	1.6	1.3	1.0	0.0	2.2	1.2

FUNCTIONAL HEALTH

It is useful to follow our consideration of chronic diseases and conditions with an assessment of functional health as it is associated with social class. A functional assessment of health examines the behavioral consequences of chronic disease morbidity (Longino & Soldo, 1987). Deficit functional capacities are viewed as relating directly to the need for assistance, usually from another person, in such basic activities as eating, bathing, and dressing (Katz, 1983). Such functional dependency has both an objective and a subjective component. The need for help may be emphatically denied by one person, while another person with the same physical condition may eagerly assert it. For that reason it is difficult to assess. In addition, the degree of severity of functional dependency can vary substantially from one person to another.

The decline in functional health carries with it an increase in vulnerability and dependency. When one has difficulty in eating or dressing or walking on a long-term basis, then something at the core of the individual is challenged. Self-sufficiency in these elemental areas of personal care marked passages from infancy to independent childhood. "I can do it myself" is a feeling that comes early in life, and it is a good feeling for most of our lives. Because we have been socialized to be independent in our personal care, the loss of our ability to care for ourselves makes us feel vulnerable and appear vulnerable to others. Functional health, and its decline, carries with it a psychological cost as well.

There is also a sociological dimension to functional dependency. In all societies there are some persons whose needs are met in abundance and others for whom even basic needs are not well met. Vulnerability, therefore, is a variable and comparative concept. A universal value in natural human communities, within the limits of their resources, is to care for and protect the dependent. The infant and the child receive special attention, for they are its future. The old and the incapacitated are its trust. There is even a general concern for the temporarily dependent, such as the sick and the pregnant, when resource levels are adequate. This universal human value for the care and protection of dependent people has been implemented by national social legislation as our resources as a nation state have grown. When we temporarily reached the limits of the welfare state in the early 1980s, we were called to reassess our values, our resources, and our commitments.

When economic vulnerability is added to that of health in old age, the human resources of the household and kinship network become critical since the present system of state agencies does not nearly meet the needs of older people whose capabilities are declining but who continue to live in independent households (Susser & Watson, 1971).

As early as 1959, research was demonstrating that social class was related to chronic disability among men in England. Edwards, Mc-Keown, and Whitfield (1959) compared the disability prevalence of men in three social class categories in their sixties and similarly in their seventies. These researchers were able to show that even though the prevalence of disability increased with age, the social class effect remained. Studies of social class and disability (Chirikos & Nickel, 1986) tend more often to concern themselves with work disability and its economic advantages.

Table 3.7 shows each of the items of the Activities of Daily Living Scale and selected items from the Instrumental Activities of Daily Living Scale as they are associated with the two measures of social class.

Difficulties with chewing and walking are the most frequently cited functional limitations, and both are strongly associated with social class. Over a quarter of the individuals in the lowest quartile of socio-economic status had difficulty chewing or walking. Less than a sixth

TABLE 3.7 Functional Limitations by Social Class

	Socioeconomic Quartiles				Poverty Level	
	Lowest	Second	Third	Highest	Below	Above
Percent Having Difficulty with:						
Chewing	27.5	15.6	8.8	6.5	28.1	14.3
Eating	2.4	0.7	0.8	1.1	2.4	1.3
Bathing	12.2	4.4	3.3	2.7	12.1	6.2
Dressing	8.3	3.7	2.8	2.7	8.7	4.9
Arising*	10.7	4.1	4.0	3.2	12.4	6.3
Walking	27.1	13.9	8.7	5.9	28.0	14.2
Getting Outside	14.1	4.6	3.2	3.8	15.1	6.5
Bladder Control	11.2	5.4	5.4	2.2	11.9	6.1
Percent Having Difficulty with Instrumental Activities						
Preparing Meals	8.5	3.4	2.6	2.8	9.2	4.9
Shopping	16.1	6.2	3.7	3.8	17.4	7.6
Light Housework	9.5	4.5	2.6	3.2	9.4	5.0
Percent with 1+ Functional Limitations	72.8	49.9	39.3	27.0	72.2	49.5
Personal Care(%)						
Unable to Care for Oneself	5.7	2.7	1.2	2.3	6.6	2.5
Limited Ability	12.2	4.4	3.6	2.3	12.3	4.9
No Limits	80.3	90.2	91.1	90.9	79.3	89.9
*Percent Retired Due to Health**￼*	40.5	19.7	20.1	10.1	42.4	23.7

* Getting in or out of a bed or chair.
** for those who retired.

the proportion, about six percent, of those in the highest quartile had difficulty with these activities.

Difficulty with eating is a problem for very few older persons, regardless of social class. The ability to swallow and to keep food down is the major physiologic barrier to this activity.

The other activities of daily living—bathing, dressing, getting in or out of a bed or chair, getting outside, and bladder control—show a similar pattern of association. Difficulty with each of these activities is higher among persons whose household income is below the poverty level than among economically better-off persons. The quartile measure, however, demonstrates that difficulties with these activities are concentrated in the lowest socioeconomic quartile. Differences among the second, third, and fourth quartiles are not great. Functional limitations, therefore, as measured by activities of daily living, are concentrated among the poorest segment of society.

The same pattern is seen in difficulties that some of the respondents had with the instrumental activities of daily living. Preparing meals, shopping, and light housework fell on a gradient with difficulty in each of these areas being mentioned in the highest proportions among the persons in the lowest quartile. Differences between the highest socioeconomic quartile and the next highest were negligible. Instrumental limitations are also concentrated among the least advantaged segment of the population.

Concentration of need is one thing, but the existence of need is another. When the functional limitations are combined and the question is asked, "What proportion of persons in each quartile expressed difficulty with one or more activity?," the answer obtained is found in Table 3.7. Nearly three-quarters of the national survey respondents in the lowest quartile had difficulty with at least one activity; half of those in the second quartile had some difficulty; two-fifths of the third quartile responded similarly, and just over a quarter of the respondents in the most advantaged socioeconomic quartile indicated a problem.

The Health Interview Survey included a set of questions in which the respondents were asked directly if they were able to care for themselves. Their responses were coded into three categories: no limits, limited ability, and unable to care for oneself. Eighty percent of respondents in the lowest quartile indicated that they had no limitations in their ability to handle all of their personal care by themselves; about 90 percent of the respondents in the other three quartiles gave the same total self-care response. This pattern of elevated responses in the lowest quartile confirms the patterns observed concerning activity limitations. Even though nearly three quarters of those in this quartile had indicated that they had difficulty with one or more limitation of activities, fewer than six percent said that they were unable to care for themselves and only one-eighth registered a limited ability for self-care. So, while increasing difficulty in daily activities is common among the elderly, particularly in the advanced years, the inability to care for oneself remains low, even for those in the most vulnerable socioeconomic quartile.

Those who were retired were asked if they retired due to a health problem. Forty percent of those in the lowest quartile said yes; one-fifth of the two middle quartiles and one-tenth of the highest quartile answered in like manner.

Studies of disablement in the workplace have shown (Chirikos & Nickel, 1986) that economic factors play an important role in the self-perception of functional ability. The perception of one's functional ability influences the choices governing disability-related behavior, they argue, by affecting the opportunity costs of impaired health. The economic penalties imposed by disability seem different depending on one's economic status. If one has a high-paying job, one is less likely to give it up when health is poor. Low income individuals, by contrast, are penalized less by withdrawing from work and, therefore, are more likely to be disabled. As shown in Table 3.7, the opportunity costs are more in the lowest socioeconomic quartile than in the others.

There is an accommodation process that many elderly people make to the gradual loss of capacity. In fact, 92 percent of persons 65 and over living in the community say that they have no unmet need for help with any activity of daily living, even the instrumental ones (Longino & Soldo, 1987). It is not the slowing down and reduced capacities due to arthritis or a cataract that cause the jolt to the life-style of older persons. It is the inability, or limited ability, to perform the major activities of life that is jolting. Having to stay in bed, or in a wheelchair, due to an acute illness or frailty can severely curtail one's major activities.

Table 3.8 shows that activity limitation is also related to social class. Nearly half of the persons in the lowest and nearly four-fifths of the persons in the highest socioeconomic quartile said that they had no activity limitations at all at the time of the survey. Activity limitations are more prevalent among older persons living below poverty than those living above, on all indicators. Among the poor, 17 percent were unable to perform major activities, as compared with one-tenth of those who are classified as nonpoor.

Activity limitations may respond to health fluctuations, so it is important to determine the frequency of such activity limitations. If the respondents were experiencing no activity limitations at the moment, they were asked if they had had one or more days of restricted activity in the past two weeks. One-fifth of the individuals in the lowest quartile

TABLE 3.8 Levels of Activity by Social Class

	Socioeconomic Quartiles				Poverty Level	
	Lowest	Second	Third	Highest	Below	Above
Percent with Activity Limitations						
Unable to Perform						
Major Activities	15.2	8.5	8.6	4.3	16.6	9.9
Major Activities Limited	20.1	14.1	10.6	7.0	19.7	12.8
Other Activities Limited	16.5	10.6	9.0	9.7	17.3	11.7
No Limitations	48.3	66.8	71.8	78.9	46.5	65.6
Percent with 1+ Days of Restricted Activity in Last 2 Weeks	19.8	11.5	8.7	10.8	20.5	12.0
Percent with Bed Days in Last 2 Weeks	11.1	4.4	3.8	4.9	12.4	6.0
Percent with Bed Days in Last Year						
None	57.4	67.6	67.9	65.4	55.7	64.6
1-7 Days	14.7	14.8	18.4	16.8	15.2	17.4
8-30 Days	15.6	11.1	9.2	11.9	15.1	11.6
31-180 Days	6.9	5.0	3.6	6.0	8.4	4.4
181-365 Days	3.2	1.3	0.8	0.0	3.1	1.4

had experienced such activity restrictions, as compared with half that proportion in the highest quartile.

A smaller proportion in each social class had spent a day in bed during the past two weeks. Although the association was not as strong as it was in the case of activity limitations, it was reflected mildly in bed days. Those with higher socioeconomic status more often had no days in bed during the past year.

There are services provided in the community to help older persons who need help, especially those with limitations of instrumental activities of daily living. For a person who cannot go shopping or cook meals, there is a meals program; for persons who can no longer drive and need to go to the doctor or the store, there is a transportation program. Senior centers provide a range of services as well as meeting social needs. If the poor are the most afflicted by the limitations displayed in Tables 3.7 and 3.8, then they should be the most frequent users of services aimed at meeting the needs due to these limitations

TABLE 3.9 Community Service Use by Social Class

	Socioeconomic Quartiles				Poverty Level	
	Lowest	*Second*	*Third*	*Highest*	*Below*	*Above*
Percent Using Senior Center						
Frequently	7.2	5.8	4.3	4.2	7.5	5.8
Sometimes	4.3	4.1	2.5	0.9	3.7	3.8
Rarely	2.8	3.3	3.1	2.5	3.1	3.7
Never	84.6	85.9	89.1	92.4	84.4	85.7
Percent Using Transportation Services for the Elderly						
Frequently	3.7	0.7	0.4	0.0	4.6	1.3
Sometimes	2.5	0.8	0.0	0.9	2.7	0.9
Rarely	1.0	0.8	0.2	0.0	1.1	0.8
Never	92.2	97.5	98.4	99.1	90.7	96.5
Percent Eating at Senior Center						
Frequently	5.2	2.4	1.3	1.7	5.9	2.4
Sometimes	2.5	1.5	1.7	0.9	2.5	2.2
Rarely	1.9	2.6	1.5	0.0	2.5	2.2
Never	89.2	92.5	94.4	97.5	87.8	92.4
Number of Community Services Used (%)						
About Enough	53.6	58.1	57.7	53.6	48.1	56.4
Too Much	32.7	33.1	31.7	36.4	35.0	34.1
Want to Use More	13.2	7.4	4.1	0.0	15.6	7.5

and disabilities. Table 3.9 demonstrates that service use is slight among the elderly, but lower socioeconomic status is associated with its use, as one would expect. An amusing item is the one at the foot of the table when respondents were asked if the number of community services they used were about enough, too much, or whether they wanted to use more. The bottom line again reinforces what has come to be the theme of this chapter, that the poor elderly have greater health deficits than the rich, and that they desire more services to offset their needs. The amusement, however, is with the middle line where about a third of the persons surveyed indicated that they received too much community service, although fewer than that proportion actually registered their use.

SELF-RATINGS OF HEALTH

If social class is inversely related to so many measures of chronic disease and conditions and to functional limitations, then is it reflected also in health perceptions? Is socioeconomic status associated in the same way with health perception as it is with more direct measures of health? This question is answered in Table 3.10. Respondents in the lowest socioeconomic quartile are much more likely to see themselves as having poor health than are those in the other quartiles. They are even more likely to see themselves as having fair health. In contrast, those in the highest quartile are far more likely to rate their health as excellent, and the socioeconomic association is positive among those who view themselves as being in very good health. Judging from the data contained in the other tables, this self-assessment seems realistic. Previous studies have shown self-report data from the elderly to be significantly correlated with both physician ratings and objective measures of health (Ferraro, 1980; Fillenbaum, 1979; Linn & Linn, 1980; Maddox & Douglass, 1973). These authors have gone so far as to recommend self-reports as a valid cost-effective means of health assessment (Halpert & Zimmerman, 1986). The present analysis would seem to suggest the same conclusion.

Another item in the Health Interview Survey asks respondents to evaluate their present health as compared to one year earlier. There are no differences among the socioeconomic quartiles nor among the poverty categories in the tendency of the respondents to say that their health is better. However, the better their economic position the more likely they are to say that their health has remained the same; the worse their economic position the more frequently they said that it was worse.

Two items in the survey asked the respondents to assess the level of their activity. These were also included in Table 3.10. One asked the subject to compare the amount of his activity to his peers. Even with a self-anchoring item such as this one, there is a strong social class association; the respondents from higher quartiles see themselves as more active and respondents from lower quartiles see themselves as less active than their peers.

Finally, a question was asked about participation in social activities. There was essentially no association between social class and self-assessed social participation. Between 70 and 75 percent of the individuals in all categories said that they participated in about enough

TABLE 3.10 Self-Rated Health Status by Social Class

| | Socioeconomic Quartiles | | | | Poverty Level | |
	Lowest	*Second*	*Third*	*Highest*	*Below*	*Above*
General Health (%)						
Excellent	9.0	13.8	20.9	32.4	9.7	18.6
Very Good	14.5	20.7	26.7	27.0	15.0	21.8
Good	26.2	36.0	33.3	25.4	25.1	32.0
Fair	27.8	21.2	14.5	9.7	28.2	18.6
Poor	21.8	8.2	4.1	5.4	21.4	8.6
Compared to One Year Ago (%)						
Better	10.4	11.4	12.0	10.9	12.4	12.7
Worse	23.3	11.7	8.0	12.6	23.2	11.8
Same	65.5	76.5	79.2	75.9	63.3	74.8
Amount of Activity Compared to Peers(%)						
More Active	31.3	42.5	49.1	56.9	30.9	44.7
Less Active	17.8	11.0	8.3	7.5	19.1	10.5
Same	48.2	45.8	41.7	35.6	47.9	43.5
Participation in Social Activities (%)						
About Enough	70.2	72.9	73.6	73.0	67.2	73.2
Too Much	1.2	1.9	2.6	3.5	1.4	2.3
Wants More	27.3	24.4	23.0	23.6	30.1	23.8

social activities. Fewer than 4 percent felt that their participation level was too high and about a quarter wanted more social participation.

SUMMARY AND CONCLUSION

Relatively little is known about social class and health in old age. What we know seems to come from research in England where equity in health care is an important policy issue. This chapter began with a conceptual discussion of the relationship between age, health, and social class. Since age, health and social inequality can each mean different things, the relationship is very complex. It is also dynamic because age, health and social inequality change over time. The long-term trends are for age to extend, for health to improve, and for inequality to lessen. An assessment of this subject in another generation should have somewhat different findings and conclusions. The findings presented here show a picture of strong social class differences in health among the older population in the United States.

The data presented in this chapter were derived from the 1984 National Health Interview Survey, its Supplement on Aging, conducted by the National Center for Health Statistics in Washington. Sixteen thousand one hundred and forty-eight respondents over age 55 were interviewed in a national sample.

The demographic overview demonstrated that social class, as measured here, is strongly related to age, gender, and marital status. The lower the socioeconomic quartile, the more likely the survey respondents are to be over age 75, women and widows; young (55-64), married and male respondents tended to concentrate in the higher quartiles. This raised questions about confounding variables. How many of the differences in health that were found in this chapter were due less to social class than to gender or old age, for example? The answer is not available from the present analysis.

Mortality and social class in old age have apparently not been studied in the United States. The British studies admit to many thorny measurement problems and find relatively few social class differences in mortality rates in old age. Considering the other findings in this chapter, however, such a relationship may be found in the United States.

Disease-specific mortality rates, as related to social class in old age, have only begun to be studied. Cancer, for example, seems to have a positive association with social class. Mortality studies of the elderly will soon be possible, using the new data set called the Longitudinal Study of Aging, produced beginning in 1987 by the National Center for Health Statistics. It will link mortality data from the National Death Registry to the health records as soon as the respondents die.

Major disease prevalence is not uniformly related to social class. Heart disease is apparently not related at all, cancer is positively related, and stroke is negatively related.

Other less deadly chronic diseases and conditions are often negatively related to social class. This is so in the adult population over age 17, and equally so among the elderly. The lower the social class, the higher the prevalence of heart condition, hypertension, diabetes, varicose veins, arthritis, and vision and hearing impairment. There are no social class differences, however, in the use of health care services.

The same negative association with social class is found for nearly every measure of functional health: ADL, IADL difficulties, the need for personal care, retirement due to health problems, activity limitations, and community services. Self-ratings of health follow the same pattern. The poor think they are less healthy, and it seems that they are right.

Few older people use community services, but, of those who do, the economically disadvantaged seem to use them more and want more services than other older persons.

This analysis is only a first step in the study of age, health, and social class. It cracks the door, but only slightly. First, studies that follow should simultaneously control for the effect of age, gender, and marital status so that a clearer picture of the effect of social class on health will result. The demographic overview demonstrates the necessity for this step.

Second, more general mortality studies would be extremely useful. Marmot (1986) found that there are important mortality SES differences between British civil servants approaching retirement. This suggests that the likely hypothesis is easier to come by than the necessary measures of socioeconomic status. It is an issue that needs some research attention.

Third, as suggested above, the LSOA data set from NCHS should be ideal for studying major causes of death by social class among the elderly. By 1990 there should be enough accumulated cases to make an exploratory study worthwhile.

Fourth, it would be worthwhile to assess the accuracy of health self-ratings for the social class categories in old age. Do chronic diseases and conditions predict self-assessment better than functional health, and do they predict differently for the economically advantaged and disadvantaged? The Supplement on Aging of the National Health Interview Survey would provide an appropriate data set for such a study.

Finally, an assessment of the relative proportion of the variance attributable to gender and social class would be most useful. Social class differences may not be as great when separated by gender as one might suppose since there is little evidence that class and health vary by gender. Such a study, however, would bridge the two chapters on these separate subjects in this book.

REFERENCES

Barsky, A. J. (1988). The paradox of health. *New England Journal of Medicine, 318*, 414-418.

Berkman, L. F., & Breslow, L. (1983). *Health and ways of living: The Alameda County study*. New York: Oxford University Press.

Branch, L. G., & Jette, A. M. (1984). Personal health practices and mortality among the elderly. *American Journal of Public Health, 74*, 1126-1129.

Chirikos, T., & Nickel, J. T. (1986). Socioeconomic determinants of continuing functional disablement from chronic disease episodes. *Social Science and Medicine, 22*, 1329-1335.

Edwards, F., McKeown, T., & Whitfield, A. G. W. (1959). Incidence of disease and disability in older men. *British Journal of Preventive Society of Medicine, 13*, 51-58.

Ferraro, K. F. (1980). Self-ratings of health among the old and the old-old. *Journal of Health and Social Behavior, 21*, 377-383.

Fillenbaum, G. G. (1979). Social context and self-assessment of health among the elderly. *Journal of Health and Social Behavior, 20*, 45-51.

Fox, A. J., Goldblatt, P. O., & Jones, D. R. (1986). Social class mortality differentials: Artefact, selection, or life circumstances. In R. G. Wilkinson (Ed.), *Class and Health.* New York: Tanstock.

Guralnick, L. (1967). Selected family characteristics and health measures reported in the Health Interview Survey. *Vital and Health Statistics, 1000*, 6.

Halpert, B. P., & Zimmerman, M. K. (1986). The health status of the "old-old": A reconsideration. *Social Science and Medicine, 22*, 893-899.

Kaplan, G. A., Haan, M. N., Syme, S. S., Minkler, M. M., & Winkleby, M. (1987). Socioeconomic status and health. In R. W. Amler and H. B. Dull (Eds.), *Closing the gap: The burden of unnecessary illness*. New York: Oxford University Press.

Kart, C. S. (1985). *The realities of aging*. Newton, MA: Allyn and Bacon.

Katz, S. (1983). Assessing self-maintenance: Activities of daily living, mobility and instrumental activities of daily living. *Journal of American Geriatric Society, 31*, 721-727.

Kitagawa, E. M. (1969). *Social and economic differentials in mortality in the United States, 1960.* Paper presented at the General Assembly and Conference of International Union for Scientific Study of Population, London.

Kitagawa, E. M., & Hauser, P. M. (1968). Education differentials in mortality by cause of death, United States, 1960. *Demography, 5*, 340.

Linn, B. S., & Linn, M. W. (1980). Objective and self-assessed health in the old and very old. *Journal of Health and Social Behavior, 14*, 311-315.

Longino, C. F., Jr. (1987a). *The Social and economic characteristics of very old men and women in the United States.* Paper presented at the annual scientific meeting of the Gerontological Society of America, Washington, DC.

Longino, C. F., Jr. (1987b). *What else kills older Floridians? Non-cancer rates by cause of death in Florida counties among age, race and sex categories.* Coral Gables, FL: University of Miami, Center for Social Research in Aging.

Longino, C. F., Jr. (1988). Who are the oldest Americans? *The Gerontologist, 28*, 515-523.

Longino, C. F., Jr., & Soldo, B. (1987) The graying of America: Implications of life extension for quality of life. In R. A. Ward & S. S. Tobin (Eds.), *Health and aging: Sociological issues and policy directions* (pp. 58-85). New York: Springer.

Longitudinal Study of Aging. (1986). The National Center for Health Statistics, DHHS. Washington, DC: U.S. Government Printing Office.

Maddox, G. J., & Douglass, E. B. (1973). Self-assessment of health: A longitudinal study. *Journal of Health and Social Behavior, 14*, 87-93.

Markides, K. S., & Machalek, R. (1984). Selective survival, aging and society. *Archives of Gerontology and Geriatrics, 3*, 202-222.

Marmot, M. G. (1986). Social inequalities in mortality: The social environment. In R. G. Wilkinson (Ed.), *Class and health.* New York: Tanstock.

Minkler, M., & Stone, R. (1985). The feminization of poverty and older women. *The Gerontologist, 25*, 351-357.

Palmore, E. (1978). When can age, period and cohort be separated? *Social Forces, 57*, 282-295.

Palmore, E. (1986). Trends in the health of the aged. *The Gerontologist, 26*, 298-302.

Riley, M. W. (1987). On the significance of age in sociology: American Sociological Association 1986 presidential address. *American Sociological Review, 52*, 1-14.

Soldo, B. J., & Longino, C. F., Jr. (1988). Social and physical environments of the vulnerable aged. In M. P. Lawton & W. Bell (Eds.), *A social and built environment for an aging society.* Washington, DC: National Academy Press.

Soldo, B. J., & Manton, K. G. (1985). Demographic challenges for socioeconomic planning. *Socioeconomic Planning Science, 19*, 227-247.

Susser, M. W., & Watson, W. (1971). *Sociology in medicine.* London: Oxford University Press.

Verbrugge, L. M. (1984). Longer life but worsening health? Trends in health and mortality of middle-aged and older persons. *Milbank Memorial Fund Quarterly/Health and Society, 62*, 475-519.

Verbrugge, L. M. (1987). From sneeze to adieux: Stages of health for American men and women. In R. A. Ward & S. S. Tobin (Eds.), *Health in aging: Sociological issues and policy directions.* New York: Springer.

Wilkinson, R. G. (1986a). *Class and health.* New York: Tanstock.

Wilkinson, R. G. (1986b). Income and mortality. In R. G. Wilkinson (Ed.), *Class and health.* New York: Tanstock.

CHAPTER 4

Physical Health Conditions of Middle-Aged and Aged Blacks

JACQUELYNE JOHNSON JACKSON
CHARLOTTE PERRY

INTRODUCTION

Our primary focus on differences by age, sex, and marital status in the physical health conditions of middle-aged and aged blacks in the United States begins with descriptions of their aggregated demographic and health conditions. The discussion of these differences within the context of the ethnogerontologic and related literature emphasizes research gaps about the determinants of the health conditions of black cohorts as they age.

Unless otherwise noted, *middle-aged* and *aged* persons, respectively, are between age 40-64 years and 65 or more years. The demographic data include recent population estimates, usually by sex and age, of education, income, employment, marital status, living arrangements, and perceptions of neighborhood conditions and services. Health indicators include death rates for all causes of death and major causes of death, morbidity rates for acute and chronic diseases, and rates of disability, limitation of activity, and respondent-assessed and self-reported health status. Some of these data are supplemented by black and white comparisons.

The major sources of data are the U.S. Bureau of the Census, National Center for Health Statistics, National Cancer Institute, and post-1966 ethnogerontologic and related publications. Fiscal limitations prevented an exhaustive search of the literature and use of public data tapes, but most of the available literature was examined.

TABLE 4.1 Percentage Distributions of the Total Black Population, by Sex and Age, and Sex Ratios, United States, 1986 and 1980 (numbers in thousands)

AGE (in years)	Females 1986	Females 1980	Males 1986	Males 1980	Sex Ratios 1986	Sex Ratios 1980
# all ages	15,917	14,538	15,234	13,934	95.7	95.8
% Under 40	69.6	70.1	73.2	73.3	99.3	100.2
%40-44	5.3	5.0	5.3	5.0	94.9	96.0
%45-49	4.7	4.6	4.6	4.6	94.1	95.8
%50-54	4.1	4.4	4.0	4.3	93.4	94.1
%55-59	3.9	4.0	3.7	3.8	90.9	90.0
%60-64	3.5	3.4	3.1	3.0	86.0	84.7
%65-69	2.8	2.9	2.3	2.3	79.1	77.1
%70-74	2.3	2.2	1.7	1.7	69.3	71.7
%75-79	1.7	1.6	1.1	1.0	61.0	63.4
%80-84	1.1	1.0	0.6	0.6	52.2	56.2
%85+	1.0	0.8	0.5	0.4	41.0	45.8
%40-64	21.4	21.4	20.6	20.7	92.3	92.7
%65+	9.0	8.5	6.2	6.0	65.4	67.6

SOURCE: Raw data from U.S. Bureau of the Census, 1987(a), Table A-1.

Four major assumptions about blacks and whites in the United States are that (1) blacks have no unique or peculiar health conditions, (2) the aging of blacks and whites of similar socioeconomic and environmental conditions is more similar than dissimilar, (3) the significant variations between black and white health conditions are best explained by racism and differential environmental conditions, and (4) blacks are not genetically inferior to whites.

DEMOGRAPHIC OVERVIEW

Population Estimates and Sex Ratios

Table 4.1 contains population estimates (adjusted for the net census undercount) and percentage distributions by sex and age of the total black population in the United States in 1980 and 1986, and their sex ratios (the number of males per 100 females) and component changes.

The population increase between 1980 and 1986 of each sex-age group was generally highest among the youngest middle-aged and the three oldest groups. The percentages of middle-aged and aged persons in each sex group remained relatively constant. About 30 percent of the females and 26 percent of the males in each year were middle-aged or aged.

The sex ratio of blacks under age 40 years was about equal. Female preponderance among the middle-aged and aged increased with age. The largest increases between 1980 and 1986 of female preponderance among the four oldest groups reflect the growing longevity gaps between women and men.

Education

Table 4.2 generally shows increased educational levels between 1980 and 1987 of middle-aged and aged blacks of each sex, and no gender differences in the average educational levels of persons at age 25 or more years and 40-54 years. The increased educational level and percentages of high school and college graduates among middle-aged and aged blacks generally followed the usual pattern of inverse relationship between education and age.

Unlike the decrease between 1980 and 1987 in the educational level among black men at age 70-74 years, the slight decrease between 1980 and 1987 is quite slight. These shifts, as well as proportionately fewer college graduates among aged blacks of both sexes, may be due to the changing influences of education on longevity. Medicare and Medicaid have helped improve access to mainstream health care among adults of all educational levels. By the turn of the century, the vast majority of native-born, middle-aged blacks will probably be high school graduates, but not college graduates.

The increase between 1980 and 1987 in average education among the cohorts for whom such data were available are probably best explained by higher mortality among their more poorly educated than better educated members. These kinds of data may reflect a continuing weakening of the historical pattern of substantially positive correlations between black mortality and education.

Table 4.2 Educational Levels of Blacks, 25+ Years of Age, by Sex and 40+ Years of Age, by Sex and Age, United States, 1980 and 1987

Age	Women		Men	
	1987	*1980*	*1987*	*1980*
Median years of school completed				
25+ years of age	12.4	12.0	12.2	12.0
40-44 years of age	12.5	12.2	12.5	12.2
45-49 years of age	12.4	11.9	12.4	11.3
50-54 years of age	12.2	10.9	12.1	10.5
55-59 years of age	11.6	10.1	10.5	9.5
60-64 years of age	11.7	8.7	9.6	8.7
65-69 years of age	10.2	8.4	8.7	7.8
70-74 years of age	8.9	7.9	7.5	7.6
75-79 years of age	—	4.8	—	4.8
75+ years of age	7.9	—	6.7	—
% High school graduates				
40-64 years of age	37.3	28.1	28.4	26.0
65+ years of age	16.9	11.1	13.4	11.3
% College graduates				
40-64 years of age	7.5	4.5	9.8	3.2
65+ years of age	6.0	3.7	4.3	8.3

SOURCE: U.S. Bureau of the Census, 1988, Table 2, and U.S. Bureau of the Census, 1984(a), Table 2.

Income and Employment

Table 4.3 shows the median total money income of all blacks and black year-round, full-time workers, at age 40 or more years, by sex and age, in the United States in 1982 and 1985 (in constant 1985$). The income levels of all women and men, as well as of employed women and men, generally decreased with increasing age. With the sole exception of all women at age 60-64 years, the median income of all women and employed women rose between 1982 and 1985. Only the 60-64-year-olds among all men had less income in 1985 than in 1982. In contrast, the median income for most of the age groups among employed men fell between 1982 and 1985. The gaps by sex between all women and all men were generally greater than those between employed women and employed men.

Table 4.3 Median Total Money Income of All Blacks and Black
Year-Round, Full-Time Workers, Age 40+ Years, by Sex
and Age, United States, 1985 and 1982 (in constant 1985$)

Characteristic, Sex & Year	Age (in years)						
	40-44	45-49	50-54	55-59	60-64	65-69	70+
All women							
1985 ($)	11,310	10,553	9,524	6,935	4,396	4,495	4,420
1982 ($)	9,232	8,701	8,283	6,881	5,179	4,308	3,038
Employed women							
1985 ($)	16,113	15,660	15,236	14,913	13,798	(B)	(B)
1982 ($)	15,061	12,786	14,102	13,188	11,895	(B)	(B)
All men							
1985 ($)	17,988	18,128	15,972	12,724	9,414	7,215	6,140
1982 ($)	15,867	14,558	14,008	8,955	12,076	6,538	5,468
Employed men							
1985 ($)	18,512	18,458	17,512	17,473	16,696	(B)	(B)
1982 ($)	19,108	18,411	18,908	18,439	19,241	(B)	(B)

SOURCES: U.S. Bureau of the Census, 1984(c), Table 46, and U.S. Bureau of the Census, 1987(c), Table 34.

(B) = base less than 75,000 prevents reliable estimate.

As expected, most aged women and men who were employed in
1982 and 1985 were not year-round, full-time workers. Striking, however, is the fact that most employed black middle-aged women and men
in those two years were not year-round, full-time workers.

The changing labor force patterns of middle-aged and aged blacks
are also reflected in their rising unemployment levels between 1972
and 1985 (see U.S. Department of Labor, 1985, 1986). Comparisons of
seven-year annual averages of black female and male unemployment
rates show substantial increases among women at ages 35-44 years
(22.1%), 45-54 years (41.5%), 55-64 years (24.4%), and 65 or more
years (59.4%). Generally greater increases occurred among men at ages
35-44 years (74.1%), 45-54 years (53.7%), 55-64 years (61.2%), and 65
or more years of age (32.3%). The typically higher male than female
unemployment rates represent a rather strong reversal of the historic
pattern of typically higher black female than male unemployment rates
(Jackson, 1973b).

Table 4.4 Seven-Year Annual Averages of Black Unemployment Rates, Age 35 or More Years of Age, by Sex and Age, United States, 1972-1978 and 1979-1985, and Component Changes

	1979-1985 Age (in years)				1972-1978 Age (in years)				% Change, 1979-1985/1972-1978 Age (in years)			
Sex	*35-44*	*45-54*	*55-64*	*65+*	*35-44*	*45-54*	*55-64*	*65+*	*35-44*	*45-54*	*55-64*	*65+*
Women	9.4	7.5	5.6	5.1	7.7	5.3	4.5	3.2	22.1	41.5	24.4	59.4
Men	10.1	8.3	7.9	8.6	5.8	5.4	4.9	6.5	74.1	53.7	61.2	32.3

SOURCES: U.S. Department of Labor, Bureau of Labor Statistics, 1986, Table 3; 1985(a), Table 3; and 1985(b), Table 27.

These unemployment rates help to explain, but not entirely, the perennially much higher black than white poverty rates of either sex. The poverty rates of black and white women and men 35 or more years of age in 1985 fit the expected pattern and may be seen only for blacks in Table 4.4. In addition, despite the tremendous decrease since 1959 in both the aged black and white poverty rates, the annual black-to-white ratio has actually widened: from 1.8882 in 1959 to 2.8636 in 1985 (Jackson, 1987).

Marital Statuses

Earlier analyses of changes in adult black marital statuses and comparative adult black and white marital statuses since 1960 (Jackson, 1973b, 1980, 1985) have shown both rising proportions of never married blacks (generally higher among males) and racially widening gaps by sex that are particularly pronounced among young and middle-aged adults. Six-year annual averages between 1979 and 1984 of the percentage distributions of black and white marital statuses of persons at age 25 or more years (Table 4.5) show that spousal absence caused by separation, widowhood, or divorce is higher in each age group among black women than among white women, black men, and white men. Most black women in each age group shown in Table 4.5 were not then married *and* living with husbands. Spousal absence by sex among blacks and whites was more pronounced among the women than among the men.

Households and Families

Of the estimated 9,797,000 black households in the United States in 1986, 84.4 percent were in metropolitan areas and 52.7 percent were in the South, as were 54.1 percent of all black household members, 41.4 percent of whom were, or resided with, female householders. About 55.3 percent of all black householders in 1986 were also middle-aged or aged (U.S. Bureau of the Census, 1987e).

The household and family characteristics of middle-aged and aged blacks in the United States in 1986 (Table 4.6) generally show inverse relationships between age of householder and family households with married couples or female heads. Conversely, the proportion of non-family households, including those of female householders, rises with age.

Table 4.5 Six-Year Annual Averages of Percentage Distributions of Black and White Marital Statuses, 25+ Years of Age, by Sex and Age, United States, 1979-1984

	Age Group (in years)					
Sex and Marital Status	*25-34*	*35-44*	*45-54*	*55-64*	*65-74*	*75+*
Black Women	32.1	13.0	8.1	5.8	4.2	4.6
% Never married	40.6	48.9	47.8	43.7	33.1	14.6
% Married with spouse	14.3	16.0	15.0	11.2	7.0	3.2
% Married, spouse absent	1.2	4.9	13.6	28.6	49.8	74.4
% Widowed	11.8	17.2	15.6	10.7	5.9	3.2
% Divorced						
Black Men	37.7	15.0	11.4	6.8	5.6	4.0
% Never married	47.8	59.9	61.3	63.0	64.4	52.3
% Married with spouse	6.9	10.8	10.9	11.9	8.3	6.5
% Married, spouse absent	0.2	1.0	4.4	8.2	16.0	32.8
% Widowed	7.3	13.4	12.0	9.9	5.7	4.4
% Divorced						
White Women	15.0	5.0	4.0	4.2	5.5	6.4
% Never married	70.9	78.1	77.8	69.8	49.9	23.0
% Married with spouse	3.9	3.6	3.0	2.1	1.4	1.0
% Married, spouse absent	0.6	1.8	5.9	16.9	38.7	67.4
% Widowed	9.6	11.5	9.2	7.0	4.6	2.2
% Divorced						
White Men	24.9	7.9	5.4	4.9	5.2	3.8
% Never married	65.2	80.6	83.9	85.1	81.6	70.4
% Married with spouse	2.8	2.8	2.5	1.9	1.7	1.7
% Married, spouse absent	0.3	0.3	1.1	3.2	7.9	22.0
% Widowed	7.0	8.4	7.0	4.9	3.7	2.1
% Divorced						

SOURCES: U.S. Bureau of the Census (1980-1983, 1984d, and 1985a)

A much larger proportion of families with married couples than without married couples were in owner-occupied units. The reverse was true of public housing tenants. The average size of households headed by middle-aged persons was greater among married couples than among female-headed households, with the reverse being true of households with aged heads.

Table 4.6 Household and Family Characteristics of Blacks, Age 40+ Years, by Age, United States, 1986 (numbers in thousands)

| Characteristic | Age of Householder (in years) | | | | |
	40-44	45-54	55-64	65-74	75+
# All Households	843	1,680+	1,250	1,058	586
% Family households	79.7	72.1	66.2	54.2	48.0
% Married couples	43.5	40.2	42.8	35.4	25.6
% Other female householder	31.6	28.3	20.1–	15.0–	18.8
% Nonfamily households	20.3	27.9+	33.8	45.8	52.0
% Female householder	7.7	12.6+	20.9+	31.8	38.6
# Married-Couple Families	367	676+	535	375	150
Tenure					
% Owner families	69.2	77.4	82.4	78.7	76.7
% Private renters	26.4–	20.3+	14.8–	15.7	16.0
% Public housing	4.1–	2.4–	3.0–	5.3+	7.3+
Average # of members	4.49	3.83–	3.44	2.90	2.59
# Other Families, Female Householders	266	476+	251–	159–	110
Tenure					
% Owner families	40.2	50.4	60.2	64.8+	64.5
% Private renters	43.2	37.6	28.7	27.0+	26.4–
% Public housing	16.5–	12.2–	11.6	8.2–	9.1+
Average # of members	3.74–	3.87	3.31	3.41	3.22

SOURCES: U.S. Bureau of the Census, 1987(e), Tables 3 and 22, and U.S. Bureau of the Census, 1985(b), Tables 3 and 22.

+ and – show percentage increases or decreases of 10 or more points respectively between the comparative data for 1986 and 1984 (for which the data are not shown).

The household and family characteristics in Table 4.6 that increased or decreased between 1984 and 1986 by at least ten percentage points are identified by a + or – sign. Particularly striking is the significant increase in public housing tenure among the aged married couples and the very oldest families with female householders. The percentage of public housing tenure among families with female heads, at age 75 or more years, for instance, rose from 2.8 percent in 1984 to 9.1 percent in 1986. This increase may be partially explained by sampling errors, but it also probably reflects the increasing longevity of poor black women into the later stages of life, some of whom were undoubtedly public housing tenants during their earlier years.

Table 4.7 Characteristics of Housing Units Occupied by Black Householders, United States, 1983 and 1970 (numbers in thousands) and Component Changes

Characteristic	1983	1970	% Change 1983/1970
Number of all occupied units	9,163	6,174	48.4
% Inside Standard Metropolitan Statistical Areas	77.8	76.8	1.3
% in central cities	57.0	62.1	−8.2
% owner occupied	45.0	41.6	8.2
% With all plumbing facilities: owner-occupied	95.6	85.6	11.7
renter-occupied	94.7	82.4	14.9
% With complete kitchen facilities for exclusive			
use of household: owner-occupied	98.2	90.2	8.9
renter-occupied	96.4	87.6	10.0
% With no heating equipment	0.3	1.7	−82.4
% With no air conditioning	52.5	82.0	−36.0
% With no telephone	19.8	30.1	−34.2
Median number of persons in unit: owner-occupied	3.0	3.3	−9.1
renter-occupied	2.3	2.8	−17.9
Mean number of rooms: owner-occupied	5.7	5.5	3.6
renter-occupied	4.1	4.0	2.5
% 1.00 or fewer persons per room: owner-occupied	94.2	84.5	11.5
renter-occupied	91.0	77.8	4.1
Source of water			
% Public system, private company, or individual well	99.3	97.7	1.6
Sewage disposal			
% Public sewer, septic tank, or cesspool	98.0	94.4	3.8

SOURCE: U.S. Bureau of the Census, 1984b, Table A-7.

Table 4.7 displays selected characteristics of housing units occupied by black householders in the United States in 1970 and 1983 and their component changes. The substantial increase in the number of occupied units was accompanied by a slight increase in the proportion of housing units located inside Standard Metropolitan Statistical Areas (SMSA's) and a statistically insignificant decrease in the number of housing units in central cities. The percentages of black householders living in relatively new units decreased between 1970 and 1983 among owner-occupied households. The reverse was true of renter-occupied households.

Almost all of the occupied units in 1983, most of which were built before the past two decades, had plumbing, complete kitchen, and heating facilities or equipment. Most of the units also had relatively adequate space per person and a reasonably sufficient water and sewage disposal. Very few, however, had air conditioning and almost 20 percent had no telephone.

As shown in Table 4.8, most black householders in the United States in 1983 did not perceive themselves as being bothered by adverse conditions in their neighborhoods. They were, instead, generally satisfied with their neighborhood services, including their existing hospitals or health clinics. Neighborhood dissatisfaction, however, was far more common among householders in renter-occupied than in owner-occupied units.

Demographic Traits and Health Conditions

The demographic descriptions presented above are related to or influence in varying ways the health conditions of blacks throughout their life cycles. For instance, spousal absence appears to be indirectly and inversely related to longevity among aged black women. The effects of education, income, and employment on black health attitudes and behaviors, as well as access to and use of mainstream health care facilities, have not remained constant during the past several decades. Adequate housing and neighborhood conditions and satisfaction with those conditions also impact upon black physical and mental health. For example, a middle-aged black man who has a coronary heart attack in a home that has no telephone is at much greater risk for immediate death than is his counterpart who has an operable telephone.

Unfortunately, however, most of the rates of mortality, morbidity, and functionality of middle-aged and aged blacks reported below are usually cross-tabulated only by sex and age. For instance, although longevity and socioeconomic status are inversely related, the reported death rates are not cross-tabulated by education, income, and major lifetime occupation. An important caveat here is the critical distinction between *age differences* (apparent in cross-sectional data) and *age changes* (apparent in longitudinal data). Most of the ethnogerontologic and related literature on black health conditions focuses on *age differences* and not on *age changes*. Age differences do not provide any data

Table 4.8 Perceptions of Neighborhood Conditions and Services and Overall Opinions of Neighborhood of Black Householders in Owner-Occupied and Renter-Occupied Housing Units, United States, 1983

Characteristic	Owner-Occupied			Renter-Occupied		
		Inside SMSAs			*Inside SMSAs*	
	Total	*Rural*	*Urban*	*Total*	*Rural*	*Urban*
Neighborhood Conditions						
% With bothersome:						
street or highway noise	11.4	10.4	12.1	14.3	14.8	15.8
streets needing repair	16.5	19.9	11.5	10.1	18.8	11.0
commercial or nonresidential activities	2.0	2.0	2.6	2.5	1.0	3.0
odors, smoke, or gas	6.2	9.0	6.7	6.7	5.0	8.2
neighborhood crime	9.4	11.4	14.8	10.2	11.9	16.5
trash, litter, or junk	12.8	12.4	16.8	11.4	5.0	17.0
boarded-up or abandoned structures	4.8	2.5	6.2	3.9	1.0	6.2

Neighborhood Services

% With unsatisfactory:						
police protection	9.9	10.0	6.7	6.5	10.9	11.2
outdoor recreation facilities	39.2	46.3	26.4	33.5	47.5	27.4
hospitals or health clinics	12.6	15.4	9.9	11.8	15.8	10.0
public transportation or none in area	52.7	31.8	9.1	38.4	66.3	17.6
neighborhood shopping	19.6	20.9	13.7	13.5	18.8	11.4
public elementary school among persons with 1 or more children in such school	4.4	4.4	4.0	4.8	2.5	5.2
Overall Opinion of Neighborhood						
% Excellent	23.5	14.7	26.5	14.7	18.8	15.3
% Good	51.2	50.0	50.7	47.9	53.5	44.4
% Fair	23.2	21.5	23.4	32.1	25.7	35.1
% Poor	2.2	2.5	2.4	5.1	2.0	5.2

SOURCE: U.S. Bureau of the Census, 1985a, Table D-14. The percentage computations excluded "not reported" or "unknown" cases.

about the aging processes and patterns of individual and population cohorts.

DEATH RATES

The major foci of this section on middle-aged and aged death rates in the United States present and compare (1) six-year annual averages between 1967 and 1984 of black and white death rates from all causes of death and black-to-white ratios, by sex and age, (2) six-year annual averages between 1979 and 1984 of ratios of black death rates by marital status, sex, and age, and (3) six-year annual averages between 1967 and 1984 by sex and age of the leading causes of black deaths.

Black and White Death Rates, All Causes of Death

The six-year annual averages of black and white age-adjusted death rates between 1967 and 1984 in the United States, as well as age-specific death rates among persons at age 40 to 85 or more years and black-to-white ratios by age and sex, shown in Table 4.9, permit cross-sectional, but not longitudinal comparisons of the data.

Mortality improvement by age-adjusted death rates in each race-sex group between the first and last time period was highest among black females (25.2%) and lower and similar among white males (18.9%), black males (18.7%), and white females (18.2%). The rank order of these age-adjusted death rates at each time period was consistently higher among black males, followed in descending order by white males, black females, and white females. The pattern of higher death rates among white males than among black females has been apparent for several decades.

Excepting black women and men at age 80-84 years, the age-specific death rates of the successively same-age cohort of each race-sex group generally declined across time. The black-to-white ratios by sex of the same-age group failed to decrease consistently across time among women at age 45-49 years and 75 or more years, as well as among men at age 45 or more years. Racial gaps by sex are usually higher, but not consistently so, among middle-aged and aged men than among their female counterparts.

Black Death Rates and Marital Status, 1979-1984

Table 4.10, based on Table 4.5, shows the death rate ratios of the various comparative pairs of marital statuses. The married deceased are not disaggregated at time of death by spousal presence or absence. Ratios higher and lower than one show higher or lower death rates respectively for the first-named marital status in the table. The never married-to-married ratio of 1.7955 of women at age 55-64 years, for instance, indicates a death rate almost 80 percent higher among the never marrieds than among the marrieds. Based on chi-square tests, the only four statistically insignificant ratios were for never married-to-widowed women at age 35-44 years and 45-54 years, never married-to-divorced men at age 25-34 years, and widowed-to-divorced men at age 45-54 years.

Unlike the significant relationships between rising death rates and age, which are apparent in each race-sex group in Table 4.10, there are only three such relationships by sex between the 12 paired marital statuses and ages shown in that table. Specifically, significant relationships exist between paired marital ratios and age for never married-to-married women, as well as men, and married-to-widowed men.

In contrast as well to the consistent pattern of significantly lower death rates for all causes of death among black married than among unmarried women or men, variations arise in similar tests of significance using black six-year annual averages of cause-specific death rates by sex and age between 1979 and 1984. More specifically, the death rates were significantly higher only among never married than widowed women at age 45-54 years, and never married than divorced men at 25-34 years. The remaining differences between the various female and male marital statuses within each age group were statistically insignificant.

The above patterns were somewhat similar by sex and age for the specific causes of death of diseases of heart, malignant neoplasms, and cerebrovascular diseases, but much less so for accidents and violent deaths. The risks of death from diseases of heart, malignant neoplasms, and cerebrovascular diseases were similar for never married, married, and divorced young women and men. The most dissimilar patterns by sex were found for homicide where the rates were always significantly lower for married than for never married, widowed, and divorced men, but not so for most such women.

Findings of higher probabilities of survivorship among marrieds than unmarrieds, as well as some changes in those probabilities both as

Table 4.9 Six-Year Annual Averages of Black and White Age-Adjusted Death Rates (all ages) and Age-Specific Rates (40-85+ years), and Black-to-White Ratios, by Sex and Age, United States, 1967-1984

Rate, Age, and Year	Females			Males		
	Black	White	Ratio	Black	White	Ratio
Age-Adjusted Rate						
1967-1972	806.9	493.2	1.636	1,299.2	886.8	1.465
1973-1978	693.4	437.1	1.586	1,171.4	792.9	1.459
1979-1984	603.9	403.6	1.496	1,056.2	719.2	1.469
Age-Specific Rate						
40-44 years of age						
1967-1972	632.8	234.7	2.696	1,084.6	414.3	2.642
1973-1978	483.8	203.7	2.375	914.0	358.1	2.552
1979-1984	369.4	165.9	2.227	758.7	300.7	2.520
45-49 years of age						
1967-1972	892.2	369.9	2.412	1,503.3	683.6	2.199
1973-1978	666.2	326.2	2.042	1,318.3	602.6	2.188
1979-1984	570.0	274.1	2.083	1,129.5	498.9	2.264
50-54 years of age						
1967-1972	1,211.9	551.5	2.198	2,040.4	1,102.0	1.852
1973-1978	1,017.8	494.4	2.059	1,895.5	962.5	1.969
1979-1984	862.6	444.0	1.943	1,651.2	834.2	1.979
55-59 years of age						
1967-1972	1,697.1	819.0	2.072	2,821.3	1,757.5	1.605
1973-1978	1,410.4	748.5	1.884	2,577.2	1,523.0	1.692
1979-1984	1,254.4	685.0	1.831	2,334.7	1,328.1	1.758
60-64 years of age						
1967-1972	2,395.0	1,220.9	1.962	3,813.6	2,712.8	1.406
1973-1978	1,988.4	1,137.0	1.749	3,512.7	2,411.4	1.457
1979-1984	1,825.0	1,063.7	1.716	3,284.4	2,074.7	1.583
65-69 years of age						
1967-1972	3,340.3	1,926.1	1.734	5,058.1	4,012.6	1.261
1973-1978	2,552.8	1,670.5	1.528	4,460.9	3,568.8	1.250
1979-1984	2,424.6	1,615.7	1.501	4,288.0	3,181.9	1.348
70-74 years of age						
1967-1972	4,647.6	3,145.7	1.477	6,946.1	5,882.2	1.181
1973-1978	4,662.9	2,779.9	1.677	6,913.0	5,449.8	1.269
1979-1984	3,597.3	2,528.9	1.422	5,965.7	4,858.0	1.228

(*continued*)

Table 4.9 Continued

Rate, Age, and Year	Females			Males		
	Black	White	Ratio	Black	White	Ratio
75-79 years of age						
1967-1972	5,825.2	5,357.7	1.087	8,557.9	8,674.4	0.987
1973-1978	5,016.9	4,575.7	1.096	7,600.2	7,949.8	0.956
1979-1984	4,908.6	4,053.4	1.211	7,584.3	7,269.7	1.043
80-84 years of age						
1967-1972	7,545.4	8,937.6	0.841	10,217.2	12,674.9	0.806
1973-1978	6,454.8	7,676.8	0.841	9,130.4	11,667.3	0.783
1979-1984	7,797.9	6,958.6	1.121	11,164.1	10,946.3	1.020
85+ years of age						
1967-1972	12,112.5	17,499.5	0.692	14,663.1	20,898.3	0.702
1973-1978	11,776.5	15,269.8	0.771	14,836.4	19,162.3	0.774
1979-1984	11,618.6	14,361.3	0.809	14,812.8	18,432.4	0.804

SOURCES: 1967 rates were computed from NCHS raw data; in 1987, upon request, NCHS provided us with 1968-1984 rates from Trend B, Table 291 (September 1982) and Trend B, Table 291 (April 1986).

Table 4.10 Six-Year Annual Averages of Black Death Rates from All Causes of Death, by Marital Status, Sex, and Age, United States, 1979-1984

Marital Status and Sex		Age (in years)					
		25-34	35-44	45-54	55-64	65-74	75+
Never married-to-married:	women	1.816	1.280	1.783	1.796	2.067	1.914
	men	2.074	2.730	2.277	2.282	2.180	2.936
Never married-to-widowed:	women	0.387	0.905@	1.012@	1.105	1.334	1.138
	men	0.461	0.606	1.332	1.359	1.321	1.914
Never married-to-divorced:	women	1.296	1.561	1.443	1.365	1.409	1.350
	men	1.054@	1.511	1.258	1.463	1.098	1.826
Married-to-widowed:	women	0.213	0.707	0.568	0.615	0.645	0.595
	men	0.222	0.222	0.585	0.596	0.606	0.652
Married-to-divorced:	women	0.714	0.440	0.810	0.760	0.682	0.706
	men	0.508	0.554	0.552	0.641	0.504	0.652
Widowed-to-divorced:	women	3.346	1.725	1.426	1.235	1.057	1.190
	men	2.286	2.496	0.945@	1.076	0.831	0.954

SOURCE: NCHS, 1982-1987.
@Chi-square tests, $p < .05$.

cohorts age and within the same age groups at different time points are not new (Mergenhagen, Lee, & Gove, 1985; Ortmeyer, 1974). In a sophisticated fifteen-year longitudinal study of mortality factors among black and white men, age 55-59 years at the beginning of a study that was statistically controlled by a number of demographic variables and by employment and health status, Mott and Haurin (1985, p. 52) still found "more favorable survival prospects" among married than unmarried men, the reasons for which remained unclear. They essentially caution against uncritical acceptance of the usual explanations for higher probabilities of survivorship among the marrieds.

Most research supports much higher survivorship for all causes of death among marrieds than among unmarrieds (Mott & Haurin, 1985). But insofar as we could determine, no researchers have investigated this thesis on the basis of cause-specific deaths among blacks. Our research did uncover some statistically insignificant differences between the marital statuses of black women and men and their cause-specific and age-specific death rates.

For example, the death rates for diseases of heart among never married-to-married and married-to-divorced rates among black women and men at age 25-34 years. The death rates for malignant neoplasms were insignificant between the never married and married women and men at age 25-34 years, as well as among the married and divorced women and men at age 25-44 years. The female and male death rates for cerebrovascular diseases were also indistinguishable among persons at age 25-44 years. Gender and marital status differences by age and sex were more pronounced for deaths due to accidents, homicide, and suicide.

Unfortunately, the data needed to explain the lack of significantly higher probabilities of survivorship among marrieds than among unmarrieds are not yet available. But we suspect that the cause includes not only demographic, structural, and social psychological factors but also health attitudes and behaviors. To date, this is a major gap in the literature about the effects of marital status on cause-specific deaths among black women and men.

Major Causes of Black Deaths, 1979-1984

Although the rank orders differ somewhat by age, the three leading causes of death of black women at 40 or more years of age between 1979 and 1984 were diseases of heart, malignant neoplasms, and cerebrovascular diseases. Much more variation existed among comparable black men. The three leading causes of death among the 40-44 year olds were diseases of heart, malignant neoplasms, and homicide and legal intervention. The black male pattern among the 45-54 year olds was diseases of heart, malignant neoplasms, and accidents and adverse effects. The male pattern among those who were 55 or more years of age then duplicated the black female pattern of diseases of heart, malignant neoplasms, and cerebrovascular diseases.

The remaining leading causes of death differ somewhat by age within each sex group, as well as by sex within each age group. For example, suicide occurred as a leading cause of death only among black men who were 40-44 years of age, while atherosclerosis appeared only among women who were over 70 years of age and among men 75 or more years of age.

The ten leading causes of death in descending order among black women at age 40-49 years were (1) malignant neoplasms, (2) diseases of heart, (3) cerebrovascular diseases, (4) chronic liver disease and cirrhosis, (5) accidents and adverse effects, (6) homicide and legal intervention, (7) infectious and parasitic diseases, (8) mental disorders, (9) diabetes mellitus, and (10) pneumonia and influenza. In contrast, for instance, the ten leading causes of death among black women over 85 years of age were (1) diseases of heart, (2) cerebrovascular diseases, (3) malignant neoplasms, (4) pneumonia and influenza, (5) atherosclerosis, (6) diabetes mellitus, (7) nephritis, nephrotic syndrome, and nephrosis, (8) infectious and parasitic diseases, (9) accidents and adverse effects, and (10) mental disorders.

The ten leading causes of death in descending order among black men at age 40-49 years were (1) diseases of heart, (2) malignant neoplasms, (3) homicide and legal intervention, (4) accidents and adverse effects, (5) chronic liver disease and cirrhosis, (6) cerebrovascular diseases, (7) mental disorders, (8) pneumonia and influenza, (9) infectious and parasitic diseases, and (10) suicide. The ten leading causes of death in descending order among black men over 85 years of age were (1) diseases of heart, (2) malignant neoplasms, (3) cerebrovascular diseases, (4) pneumonia and influenza, (5) atherosclerosis, (6) nephritis, nephrotic syndrome, and nephrosis, (7) accidents and adverse effects, (8) chronic obstructive pulmonary and allied conditions, (9) infectious and parasitic diseases, and (10) diabetes mellitus.

Black middle-aged and aged death rates specifically classified by the underlying causes of death of hypertension with or without renal disease, hypertensive heart disease, or hypertensive heart and renal disease were quite low. These combined rates between 1979 and 1984 were about one percent for black men at age 40 or more years, and about five percent for black women between 40-54 years of age, and less than two percent for black women over age 55 years.

Acquired Immune Deficiency Syndrome (AIDS)

AIDS, currently affecting less than one percent of the total black population of the United States, is *not* a leading cause of black mortality and morbidity. But compared to whites, the black incidence and prevalence rates for AIDS are disproportionately high, owing partially to higher black than white rates of intravenous drug users sharing contaminated needles and to infectant infants. The Centers for Disease Control (CDC) indicated as of 1 February 1988 that blacks accounted for about 25 percent of the 51,547 reported AIDS cases in the United States. The growing number of black AIDS victims (which apparently rose by about 38 percent just between mid-1987 and 1 February 1988) warrants consideration.

Table 4.11, based on CDC data for the United States between June 1981 and mid-1987 shows the percentage distribution of six characteristics of 7,875 black male (37.6% homosexuals, 17.1% bisexuals, and 45.3% heterosexuals) and 1,453 black female AIDS victims. The female data were not reported by sexual preference.

Fumenton (1987) has shown that the proportion of heterosexuals among black males with AIDS is artificially high inasmuch as the

> CDC originally classified the recently arrived Africans and Haitians as a separate category unto themselves, because it appeared that the disease was following a different pattern in their native countries from that in the United States. As the classification turned into a stereotype, however, the Haitian government lobbied the National Institutes of Health (NIH), a subunit of the U.S. Public Health Service, to "redesignate" this category. At first the Haitian-African groups were shifted to the cases labeled "undetermined." But in July 1986 CDC arbitrarily placed them into the heterosexual category—despite strong evidence that many of the Haitians probably acquired the illness homosexually and that much of the transmission among Africans was also not attributable to heterosexual activity. (p. 25)

This arbitrary classification among black males of foreign-born homosexuals and bisexuals as heterosexuals undoubtedly accounts for

Table 4.11 Characteristics of AIDS Victims Among Black Males (by Homosexuals, Bisexuals, and Heterosexuals) and Black Females, United States, 1981-Mid-1987

Characteristic	Black Males Homosexuals	Black Males Bisexuals	Black Males Heterosexuals	Black Females
Age at diagnosis of first AIDS disease				
Number	2,960	1,347	3,568	1,453
% Less than 12 years	0.0	0.0	0.0	9.5
% 13-29 years	31.0	30.1	17.9	29.8
% 30-39 years	45.5	41.4	52.5	45.1
% 40-49 years	16.7	19.7	18.1	10.8
% 50+ years	6.8	8.9	7.5	4.8
Time period of first diagnosis				
Number	2,960	1,347	3,568	1,453
% Before 1982	1.0	0.9	1.0	1.0
% 1982-1983	9.8	10.4	12.7	10.2
% 1984-1985	40.5	37.4	42.2	39.4
% 1986-1987	48.7	51.3	44.1	49.4
Multiple risk factors				
Number	2,960	1,347	3,426	1,315
% Only one risk factor	95.9	89.7	77.8	78.2
% Two or more risk factors	4.1	10.3	22.2	21.2
Deaths				
Number	2,960	1,347	3,568	1,453
% Not known dead	39.8	40.6	38.0	36.8
% Reported dead	60.2	59.4	62.0	63.2
Country of birth				
Number	2,960	1,347	3,426	1,453
% United States	96.6	95.1	83.5	88.7
% Haiti or Central Africa	1.0	1.4	14.6	9.4
% Other foreign country	2.3	3.5	1.8	1.9
Region of Residence				
Number	2,940	1,336	3,415	1,301
% Northeast, SMSAs	33.8	28.7	52.6	57.4
% Central, SMSAs	9.4	10.9	3.0	2.2
% West, SMSAs	16.3	13.5	3.4	2.6
% South, SMSAs	10.6	10.6	10.5	13.7
% Mid-Atlantic, SMSAs	16.1	17.2	4.7	5.1
% Not in SMSAs	13.9	19.1	25.7	21.7

SOURCE: Public use tape, Centers for Disease Control (1987), where SMSAs = standard metropolitan statistical area. Numbers less than 2,960 homosexuals, 1,347 bisexuals, and 3,568 heterosexuals among males and 1,453 among females are due to missing data on the public use tape.

their significantly larger representation among heterosexuals than among homosexuals or bisexuals.

The four groups of black homosexuals, bisexuals, male heterosexuals, and females were remarkably similar by modal age at diagnosis (i.e., 30-39 years) and time of first diagnosis (i.e., 1985-1987), presence of only one risk factor (e.g., homosexuality or intravenous drug abuser), death (i.e., mostly dead), American nativity, and modal residence (i.e., Northeastern). Chi-square results set at the alpha level of .05, however, showed statistically significant differences between black females and all black males combined only by age, nativity, and residence.

The disproportionately higher percentage of blacks in the total number of reported AIDS cases of all races between 1981 and mid-1987 was much greater among females (51.7%) than among males (22.3%). The black AIDS sex ratio during that time of 542.0 males per every 100 females was much lower than the white sex ratio of 2,866.7. Chi-square results set at the alpha level of .05 of black and whites by each variable shown in Table 4.11 (with nativity dichotomized as American-born and foreign-born) were usually statistically significant. Black and white females, as well as black and white male heterosexuals, differed significantly by each variable. Black and white bisexuals were statistically indistinguishable only by nativity, and black and white homosexuals only by nativity and time period of first diagnosis. The significant differences by race generally showed that the average black was younger by age at diagnosis, was diagnosed more recently, had higher rates of multiple risk factors, deaths, and foreign-born persons, and greater geographical concentration.

Demographic Differences in Mortality

Black death rate trends for all causes of death and most specific causes of death between 1967 and 1984 tend to be directionally similar, but magnitudiously dissimilar by such demographic variables as sex, age, and marital status. As expected, the death rates of each sex rose with age. Except for diabetes mellitus, the male rates for both all causes of death and the ten leading causes of death were always higher than the comparable female rates. This gender differential, far more pronounced among middle-aged than aged blacks, widened between 1967 and 1984 in each age-specific group. The only successive female or male cohorts whose death rates did not fall between 1967 and 1984 were those of 80- to 84-year-old black women and men and black men over 85 years of age. Mortality improvement by successive cohorts was also more pronounced among black women than among black men.

Comparisons of the rank order and the magnitude of the leading causes of death among black middle-aged and aged women and men are also associated in varying degrees with age. As age increases, a larger proportion of all deaths are attributed to fewer causes. For example, between 1979-1984, heart disease, malignant neoplasms, and cerebrovascular diseases accounted for 54.0 percent of the deaths of black women at age 40-44 years, but 71.2 percent of the deaths of black women over 85 years of age.

When compared only by race (Table 4.9), the racial ratios of age-specific death rates in each sex-age group also reveal well-established differences. These death rates are usually higher among blacks, but the magnitudes of these ratios differ considerably by sex and age, as does the pattern of the apparent racial crossover in mortality. Race alone, however, does not explain the black and white variations in death rates (Jackson, 1988).

Kitagawa and Hauser (1973), among the first to investigate systematically and comprehensively various associations between black mortality and socioeconomic variables, reported inverse relationships between them. Reid and his colleagues (1977, p. 115) indicated hyperbolically that, "It is by now well established that education is more than a way of social advancement; it is, in fact, a matter of life and death and for no group is this truer than for blacks." That generalization, however, was not based on age-specific data. The well-established relationships between mortality and marital status (see, e.g., Ortmeyer, 1974) also seem to apply to blacks (see e.g., Reid, Lee, Jeddicka, & Shin, 1977) as does Christensen's (1988) conclusion that getting married and staying married is favorably related to health status, and whose literature review showed lower rates of mortality, morbidity, disability, and mental disorders among married than among single, separated, divorced, or widowed persons.

Fortunately, the U.S. National Longitudinal Mortality Study (NLMS), a prospective study of mortality designed to "investigate socioeconomic, demographic, and occupational differences in mortality within the United States" (U.S. Department of Health and Human Services, 1988, p. 1) contains some follow-up data for 1979-1981 that shed light on these associations among blacks.

Tables 4.12 and 4.13 show NLMS standardized mortality ratios (SMRs) of black females and males by age at the start of the follow-up

Table 4.12 Mortality Ratios of Black Females in the U.S. National Longitudinal Mortality Study, 1979-1981 Follow-Up, by Age, Sex, and Other Demographic Variables

Variable	All Ages	35-44	45-54	55-64	65-74	75-84	85+	25-64	65+
All causes of death	129	180	208	138	106	104	99	—	104
Heart Disease	129	—	252	165	120	83	117	—	105
Cerebrovascular Diseases	139	—	—	—	101	165	64	—	115
Cancer	102	29	192	109	87	82	91	—	86
Lung Cancer	125	—	92	136	160	39	—	—	125
Breast Cancer	99	—	—	118	—	—	—	—	29
Geographic Divisions									
New England	119	—	152	100	—	101	—	—	—
Mid-Atlantic	109	152	125	84	111	98	77	—	99
East-West Central	94	100	92	81	85	105	101	92	95
West-North Central	132	—	—	—	—	—	—	—	156
South Atlantic	110	101	111	132	97	122	102	—	107
East-South Central	81	—	79	53	105	79	71	—	88
West-South Central	90	—	69	68	108	72	90	—	90
Mountain	63	—	—	—	—	—	—	—	—
Pacific	90	—	—	157	73	—	—	—	77
SMSA Status: Central City	106	94	112	94	119	96	102	—	108
Not in Central City	93	108	63	113	75	103	157	—	102
Not SMSA	92	112	96	107	78	103	79	—	87
Nativity: United States	99	109	105	92	103	97	99	—	100
Education (in years): 0-4	—	—	—	112	94	85	49	115	76
5-7	—	—	93	106	135	132	155	106	138
8	—	—	157	68	69	76	99	108	78

Age (in years at start of follow-up)

	(1)	(2)	(3)	(4)	(5)	(6)	(7)	(8)	(9)
High School—9-11	—	129	122	132	89	81	—	139	89
12	—	75	85	86	107	154	—	77	133
College—13-15	—	—	—	—	—	—	—	46	59
16	—	—	—	—	—	—	—	38	71
Post-Collegiate—17+	—	—	—	—	—	—	—	67	—
Family Income: Under $5,000	—	117	165	134	101	99	96	159	99
$5,000-9,999	—	146	135	108	95	81	79	114	87
$10,000-14,999	—	—	67	87	77	116	—	88	105
$15,000-19,999	—	—	104	91	—	—	—	85	155
$20,000-24,999	—	—	53	62	—	—	—	52	108
$25,000-49,999	—	—	57	46	—	—	—	37	142
Household size: One	—	—	157	121	108	80	77	138	89
Two	—	—	113	89	78	98	84	90	86
Three	—	—	117	109	97	123	—	129	109
Four	—	—	—	—	—	—	—	70	121
Five	—	—	—	—	—	—	—	91	—
Six	—	—	—	—	—	—	—	60	—
Seven	—	—	88	67	108	106	94	90	103
Marital Status: Single	—	128	85	86	—	—	—	131	114
Married	—	—	144	135	91	102	91	88	102
Separated	—	—	134	101	—	—	—	124	160
Widowed	—	—	81	77	106	94	—	109	96
Divorced	—	—	68	47	33	—	—	86	92
Employment: Employed	—	60	—	—	—	—	—	53	33
Unemployed	—	—	—	—	—	—	—	71	—
Housework	—	150	95	128	91	60	78	127	77
Unabled	—	—	—	—	220	207	144	346	186

SOURCE: U.S. Department of Health and Human Services, 1988. The mortality ratio (O/E x 100) is not shown when E is less than 5. SMSA - standard metropolitan statistical area.

Table 4.13 Mortality Ratios of Black Males in the U.S. National Longitudinal Mortality Study, 1979-1981 Follow-Up, by Age, Sex, and Other Demographic Variables

Variable	All Ages	Age (in years at start of follow-up)							
		35-44	45-54	55-64	65-74	75-84	85+	25-64	65+
All causes of death	125	197	161	156	110	83	78	—	96
Heart Disease	108	203	103	166	98	53	75	—	78
Cerebrovascular Diseases	154	—	—	—	164	91	—	—	130
Cancer	131	98	175	120	140	127	70	—	129
Lung Cancer	125	—	92	136	160	39	—	—	125
Geographic Divisions									
New England	109	—	—	—	—	—	—	—	—
Mid-Atlantic	96	62	170	63	120	61	—	—	104
East-West Central	113	132	78	106	110	168	—	—	125
West-North Central	89	—	—	116	129	—	—	—	104
South Atlantic	108	125	98	117	116	87	105	—	107
East-South Central	84	—	73	117	49	85	92	—	67
West-South Central	74	130	22	52	60	85	—	—	76
Mountain	129	—	—	—	—	—	—	—	—
Pacific	113	—	160	103	99	—	—	—	115
SMSA Status: Central City	105	111	117	89	98	131	101	—	109
Not in Central City	78	64	78	64	122	61	—	—	98
Not SMSA	104	106	78	149	90	67	109	—	86
Nativity: United States	100	99	99	103	98	101	106	—	100
Education (in years): 0-4	—	92	50	138	105	90	94	122	98
5-7	—	85	163	111	91	135	—	121	103
8	—	76	53	79	123	185	—	85	138

High School—9-11	79	108	—	62	87	105	111	—	—
12	94	94	—	—	111	92	103	—	—
College—13-15	79	70	—	—	—	48	66	—	—
16	—	70	—	—	—	—	—	—	—
Post-Collegiate—17+	—	47	—	—	—	—	—	—	—
Family Income: Under $5,000	113	155	118	105	117	159	151	143	—
$5,000-9,999	104	117	74	118	118	115	124	126	—
$10,000-14,999	79	121	—	61	87	102	161	69	—
$15,000-19,999	56	58	—	—	61	56	50	53	—
$20,000-24,999	112	67	—	—	98	76	32	102	—
$25,000-49,999	65	63	—	—	—	63	54	105	—
Household size: One	—	99	—	—	—	—	—	—	—
Two	105	88	—	—	—	137	78	115	—
Three	110	91	—	—	—	111	86	129	—
Four	89	135	—	—	139	55	146	46	—
Five	57	69	—	—	—	49	77	—	—
Six	—	127	—	—	—	—	—	—	—
Seven	99	98	—	—	101	111	94	74	—
Marital Status: Single	69	145	—	—	17	121	212	—	—
Married	92	84	107	98	87	88	82	74	—
Separated	162	112	—	—	182	79	111	—	—
Widowed	108	192	75	97	137	204	—	—	—
Divorced	124	106	—	—	125	118	109	—	—
Employment: Employed	48	57	—	37	48	43	66	61	—
Unemployed	—	107	—	—	—	79	—	—	—
Unabled	131	314	—	65	163	258	—	—	—

SOURCE: U.S. Department of Health and Human Services, 1988. The mortality ratio (O/E x 100) is not shown when E is less than 5. SMSA - standard metropolitan statistical area.

for all causes and for several specific causes of death, geographic divisions, Standard Metropolitan Statistical Area (SMSA) status, nativity only for the United States, education, family income, household size, marital status, and employment.

SMR = O/E "where O equals the observed deaths from a given cause for a characteristic of interest, and E equals the expected deaths for that cause and characteristic for a specific age-race-sex (or age-sex) group over all cohorts in the table" (U.S. Department of Health and Human Services, 1988, p. 6). The SMRs reported for the combined age-groups of 25-64 and 65 or more years of age "are age-adjusted mortality ratios using separate distributions for" each sex-age group, and therefore are "not strictly comparable between" the two sex groups (U.S. Department of Health and Human Services, 1988, p. 6). SMRs greater than or less than 100 respectively show higher observed than expected, or higher expected than observed, deaths.

Only one of the NLMS's eight cohorts included institutionalized persons, and the black sample was too small to calculate SMRs for each sex-aged group by all of the available variables. We used the *r* statistic to measure the relationship between the levels of education, income, or household size (transformed into ordinal numbers) and the SMRs in each of the two female and male age cohorts of 25-64 and 65 or more years of age, as well as the *t* statistic to test the significance of r.

Where possible to discern, the age variations in both the black female and male SMRs in Tables 4.12 and 4.13 tend to show higher observed than expected deaths among the middle-aged than the aged blacks by all causes of death, but not by each listed specific cause of death. Age variations, which also tend to be higher than expected in some geographical divisions, differ somewhat both by sex and SMSA status.

Contrary to the significantly inverse relationship between education and mortality reported by Reid and his colleagues (1977), comparisons of the SMRs of black women and men in the two age cohorts of 25-64 and 65 or more years show that the negative relationships between SMRs and education are significant within both the younger female and male cohorts, but no such relationship exists within the older female or male cohort. Thus, while more education is favorably related to mortality among the younger cohort of either sex, this advantage is not present within the older cohorts.

The inverse relationship between SMRs and income is significant only for the younger female and older male cohorts, and there are no significant relationships between SMRs and household size within any of the four cohorts of black women and men at age 25-64 years and 65 or more years.

Christensen's (1988) review stressed the advantages to health status of getting married and staying married. Our Table 4.10 also shows lower mortality rates from all causes of death among black marrieds than unmarrieds. But, contrary to Christensen's (1988) finding, being married is not always favorably related to all black cause-specific death rates in each sex-age group, a pattern most apparent for violent deaths among middle-aged and aged black women. Being married may be more favorable to male than female health, a position readily supported by Reid et al. (1977). But, granting the greater male advantage, Christensen (1988, p. 61) still emphasizes strongly that, "both sexes are clearly healthier if married than if unmarried." But these kinds of findings are challenged somewhat by the NLMS data.

The SMRs by marital status in Tables 4.12 and 4.13 show insignificant differences between being married and divorced for the younger female cohort and, perhaps surprisingly, lower than expected mortality among the widowed and divorced older females than among their remaining counterparts. The younger male cohort does not deviate from the previously reported pattern of the greater advantage of being married, but being never married is more favorable than being married within the older male cohort.

The SMRs by employment show that being employed is most favorably related to less than expected mortality, and particularly so among the older female and male cohorts. What is also striking about the age differences between the two female and male cohorts is the substantially greater SMRs for the unabled among the younger than among the older cohorts.

Other age differences between the two female and male cohorts that are apparent in the SMRs by education, family income, and household size suggest strongly that the direct or indirect effects of these various types of demographic variables are stronger within the younger than the older cohorts. These differences may reflect the unavailability of Medicare simply by age to persons under 65 years, as well as the proportionately greater Medicaid eligibility among the older than younger cohorts.

Although the prevalence of AIDS among blacks is much lower among females than males, the reported death rates from AIDS (Table 4.11) are indistinguishable by both sex and age.

Life Expectancies

Table 4.14 permits comparisons by sex and age of the average duration of life at birth, as well as the average remaining lifetime at eleven older ages, for blacks in the United States at five different time periods between 1900-1902 and 1982-1984, and component changes. The data are based on cross-sectional or current life-table methods, which, in contrast to longitudinal or generation life tables, do not reflect the mortality experience of an actual cohort from birth through death, but represent instead hypothetical cohorts. The data for the last two time periods represent three-year annual averages of the duration of lifetime or remaining lifetime for each applicable year.

The average duration of life of both sexes more than doubled between 1900-1902 and 1982-1984, with the greater improvement occurring among females. The increased life expectancy within each sex-age group was also generally more pronounced among females. The proportional increase by age among females was greater during their younger years, whereas the reverse was true of males. The occurrences of decreased life expectancies differed by sex (between 1969-1979 at ages 75 and 80 years among males, but between 1979-1981 and 1982-1984 at ages 80 and 85 years among females).

Racial Crossovers in Mortality

Although some statistical variations exist between the black and white mortality experiences in the United States during this century, the racial trends by sex are far more similar than dissimilar. But a persisting demographic and ethnogerontologic enigma is the black and white crossover in mortality. This crossover is usually measured by racial comparisons by sex of age-specific death rates, as opposed to the preferable use of probabilities of dying. The black and white crossovers in age-specific death rates and probabilities of dying are defined as the points where their curves intersect and the white rates and probabilities (previously lower than those of blacks) become and remain higher thereafter at successive ages than those of blacks. In other words, whereas the risk of death is much higher among younger blacks than whites, it is lower among very old blacks than among very old whites.

The black-to-white female and male ratios of the probabilities of dying from all causes of death in the United States between 1969-1971 and 1984 that we computed from the probabilities of death given by the

Table 4.14 Life Expectancies of Blacks, by Sex and Age and Component Changes, United States, 1900-1902 to 1982-1984

Sex and Age (in years)	Years					Percentage Change		
	1900-1902	1929-1931	1969-1971	1979-1981	1982-1984	1982-84 1900-02	1982-84 1929-31	1982-84 1969-71
Females								
At age: 0	35.0	49.5	68.3	72.7	73.6	110.3	48.7	7.8
35	27.5	30.7	37.6	40.6	41.2	49.8	34.2	9.6
40	24.4	27.5	33.3	36.1	36.7	50.4	33.4	10.2
45	21.4	24.3	29.3	31.7	32.2	50.5	32.5	9.9
50	18.7	21.4	25.5	27.4	28.1	50.3	31.3	10.2
55	15.9	18.6	22.0	23.8	24.1	51.6	29.6	9.5
60	13.6	16.3	18.7	20.2	20.5	50.7	25.8	9.6
65	11.4	14.2	15.7	16.9	17.2	50.9	21.1	9.6
70	9.6	12.2	13.0	13.7	14.1	46.9	15.6	8.5
75	7.9	10.4	10.8	11.1	11.4	44.3	9.6	5.6
80	6.5	8.6	8.9	9.1	8.8	35.4	2.3	−1.1
85	5.1	6.9	7.0	7.2	7.1	39.2	2.9	1.4
Males								
At age: 0	32.5	47.6	60.0	64.0	65.3	100.9	37.2	8.8
35	26.2	26.4	31.4	33.5	34.3	30.9	29.9	9.2
40	23.1	23.4	27.6	29.4	30.1	30.3	28.6	9.1
45	20.1	20.6	24.0	25.5	26.1	29.8	26.7	8.8
50	17.3	17.9	20.7	21.9	22.4	29.5	25.1	8.2
55	14.7	15.5	17.7	18.6	19.1	29.9	23.2	7.9
60	12.6	13.2	14.9	15.7	16.0	27.0	21.2	7.4
65	10.4	10.9	12.5	13.1	13.4	28.8	22.9	7.2
70	8.3	8.8	10.4	10.7	10.9	31.3	23.9	4.8
75	6.6	7.0	8.8	8.5	8.9	34.8	27.1	1.1
80	5.1	5.4	7.4	6.9	6.9	35.3	27.8	−6.8
85	4.0	4.3	5.9	5.3	5.5	37.5	27.9	−6.8

SOURCE: NCHS (1972, 1974, 1982-1987).

National Center for Health Statistics (1982-1987) do not support a consistent diminution of the racial gaps by sex in the probability of dying over time. Comparisons of the black and white female gaps in 1969-1971 and 1984 also show them narrowing below age 75-76 years and widening thereafter. The comparable male gaps, by contrast, widened below age 79-80 years and narrowed thereafter.

Jackson and Perry's (1988) review of the available literature on black and white crossovers in mortality in the United States showed that there were two major and competing explanations. The theoretical explanation accepts, but the methodological explanation denies the existence of the crossover. The theoretical explanation, based on the Spencerian hypothesis of "survival of the fittest," holds that the higher death rates of younger blacks than whites weed out prior to old age a substantially larger proportion of persons who are "less fit" or biologically, psychologically, and socioculturally inferior among blacks than among whites. Thus, blacks who become very old are more biologically, psychologically, and socioculturally elite than are their white counterparts. In contrast, according to the methodological explanation, the spurious crossover is based on faulty data. The use of population sizes of old blacks that were overcounted by the U.S. Bureau of the Census actually underestimates the death rates of very old blacks.

None of the literature reviewed by Jackson and Perry (1988) used a methodological approach based on generation life tables or closed populations. Such investigations could, of course, be more useful in determining definitively whether or not the reported black and white crossovers in age-specific death rates or probabilities of dying are historically real or merely artifacts of faulty data. We are generally suspicious of the accuracy of the age-specific death rates that might be or have been adjusted or reconstructed for American blacks for time periods before the past several decades. But, if there were an earlier pattern of the crossover (which can never be proven definitely), at the very least recent black and white death rates point strongly toward its disappearance.

ACUTE AND CHRONIC CONDITIONS AND RELATED OUTCOMES

There has been a substantial increase during the past few years in both the nature and amount of federally published, black-specific morbidity and related data. But, unfortunately, these data still contain very little information about the etiologic or epidemiologic relationships between or among the aging processes and health conditions of American middle-aged and aged blacks. Almost all of these largely cross-sectional data are typically cross-tabulated only by race and age or, far less often, by race, age, and sex. Many of these data are also statistically imprecise, owing largely to the inadequate sizes of black samples. In 1985, NCHS began to oversample blacks for its annual National Health Interview Survey. Even so, much of the published black data collected in 1985 are still statistically imprecise and cross-tabulated mostly by race and age only.

Another weakness of the federally published, black-specific morbidity and related data available in recent years is their lack of a relatively thorough and comprehensive coverage of the acute and chronic conditions and related outcomes among middle-aged and aged blacks in the United States. These gaps include the lack of data cross-tabulated at the very least by race, age, sex, and household or family income for the incidence, prevalence, and survival rates of their major acute and chronic conditions, as well as by degree of severity of their rates of disability and limitation of activity, use of short-stay, intermediate, and long-term health facilities, and their self-reported health assessments. Some readers might argue that this is an ill-founded criticism, owing largely to the availability of public-use tapes, including those available from NCHS. But, in addition to their relatively high costs, the use of these tapes does not resolve the problem of inadequate sizes of black samples.

Consequently the data presented below focus most heavily on published cross-sectional data where the cross-tabulations were restricted to the demographic variables of race and age or race, age and sex.

Acute Conditions

The data shown in Table 4.15 of acute conditions and related experiences among blacks at age 18-44 years and 45 or more years of age are based on estimates from NCHS's National Health Interview Survey in 1985 of the civilian, non-institutionalized population of the United States, where blacks were oversampled in an effort to improve the precision of their estimated statistics.

As expected, the number of all acute conditions reported per 100 persons in 1985 was substantially higher among the younger blacks. The two most prevalent conditions among both age groups were the common cold and influenza. Influenza occurred more often among older blacks. Most younger and older blacks received medical attention for their acute conditions, but the receipt of such attention was significantly higher among younger than older blacks.

While the number of restricted activity days and bed days associated with acute conditions was substantially greater among older blacks, there were no significant differences by age in the number of work-loss

Table 4.15 Acute Conditions, Episodes of Persons Injured, and Associated Restricted Activity Days, Bed Days, and Work-Loss Days per 100 Persons per Year of Blacks, 18-44 Years and 45 or More Years of Age, United States, 1985

Characteristic	18-44 Years of Age	45 or More Years of Age
Number of all acute conditions	130.4	98.4
% Medically attended	67.0	61.9
# of restricted activity days	723.5	862.3
# of bed days	338.6	448.9
# of work-loss days	261.3	262.2
Number of episodes of persons injured	28.4	11.5*
# of restricted activity days	363.2	470.3
# of bed days	156.2	160.1

SOURCE: NCHS, 1986a.

*The relative standard error of this statistic's numerator was > 30 percent.

days attributable to acute conditions. Injuries sustained by younger blacks were significantly higher than the number reported for older blacks, but the number of unrestricted activity days and bed days associated with injuries were much greater among older than younger blacks.

Chronic Conditions

NCHS (1986a, p. 5) defines chronic conditions "as conditions that either (a) were first noticed 3 months or more before the reference date of the interview or (b) belong to a group of conditions (including heart disease, diabetes, and others) that are considered chronic regardless of when they began." The estimated prevalence rates per 1,000 persons for 46 chronic conditions of blacks (ages 45-64, 65-74, and 75+ years) in the civilian, noninstitutionalized population of the United States in 1985 are based on data collected by NCHS (Table 4.16). The available data do not show the total number of chronic conditions per person, and data about malignant neoplasms (see Table 4.17) are excluded because these data are collected not by NCHS, but by the National Cancer Institute (NCI).

Among blacks, the reported conditions with the three highest prevalence rates per 1,000 persons differed somewhat by age. The three leading conditions of hypertension (368.4), arthritis (331.9), and sinusitis (174.7) among the 45-64 year olds may be contrasted to arthritis (581.1), hypertension (537.1), and heart disease (266.4) among the 65-74 year olds, and arthritis (577.8), hypertension (427.0), and hearing impairment (277.4) among blacks 75 or more years of age.

The three reported conditions with the highest prevalence rates among persons of all races and 18 or more years of age in the United States in 1985 are sinusitis (139.0), arthritis (128.6), and hypertension (125.1). Although there were variations by the rank ordering and magnitude of the prevalence rates, there was also considerable similarity between the most prevalent chronic conditions of the adult black and the total adult population in the United States in 1985.

Comparisons across age groups of the black-to-white ratios for each chronic condition listed in Table 4.16 show no consistent relationship with age. For example, the ratios for hypertension decrease with increasing age, whereas the ratios for hardening of the arteries increase slightly from the 45-64 year olds to the 65-74 year olds, but decline between the latter group and the oldest group. But the modal tendency of the ratios is that of decreasing black-to-white gaps with increasing age.

Cancer Incidence and Survival Rates

The second leading cause of death among black middle-aged and aged men between 1979 and 1984 was malignant neoplasms. During the same time period, cancer was the leading cause of death among black women at age 40-54 years and the second or third leading cause of death among their older counterparts. Consequently, the relatively high cancer incidence rates and relatively low survival rates among middle-aged and aged blacks are not surprising.

The age-adjusted cancer incidence rates per 100,000 for all sites combined of American black females and males between 1974 and 1983 (Table 4.17) generally rose over time. The male increase of 20.3 percent was significantly greater than the female increase of 7.1 percent. The black female-to-male ratios of the age-adjusted rates in each year show clearly that, as compared to females, the risk of cancer is much greater among males. The two highest specific cancer sites among black females during each year were breast and colon and

Table 4.16 Number of 46 Selected Chronic Conditions per 1,000 Persons, Reported in Household Interviews for Blacks, 45 or More Years of Age, by Age, in the Civilian, Noninstitutionalized Population, and Black-to-White Ratios, United States, 1985

Type of Condition	Black Rates by Age (in years)			Black-to-White Ratios by Age (in years)		
	45-64	65-74	75+	45-64	65-74	75+
Hypertension	368.4	537.1	427.0	1.491	1.292	1.085
Arthritis	331.9	581.1	577.8	1.255	1.283	1.173
Chronic sinusitis	174.7	139.2*	170.1*	0.920	0.900	1.066
Heart disease	137.0	266.4	80.8*	1.046	0.962	0.215
Hearing impairment	128.4	237.8	277.4	0.786	0.894	0.785
Deformity or orthopedic impairment	120.9	144.8	147.2*	0.738	0.624	1.197
Diabetes	112.1*	172.0	153.2*	2.458	1.686	1.708
Hay fever or allergic rhinitis	83.5	19.6*	55.5*	0.919	0.366	1.000
Trouble with corns and calluses	77.6	55.2*	61.5*	2.296	1.472	0.926
Hemorrhoids	70.4	35.0*	21.7*	0.982	0.499	0.379
Chronic bronchitis	59.3	30.8*	4.8*	1.078	0.431	0.079
Tinnitus	56.0	116.1*	65.1*	1.120	1.170	0.812
Bursitis, unclassified	51.2	84.6	32.6	1.158	2.010	1.309
Varicose veins of lower extremities	49.0	31.5*	38.6*	0.864	0.443	0.414
Visual impairments	44.9*	103.5*	78.4*	1.030	1.397	0.598
Trouble with bunions	39.7	58.0	13.3	2.295	2.479	0.314
Cerebrovascular disease	37.2*	68.5*	67.6*	2.340	1.292	1.085
Ulcer	36.6*	27.3*	51.9*	1.028	0.798	1.573
Frequent indigestion	35.9*	21.7*	55.5*	0.981	0.471	1.178
Bladder disorders	35.9*	58.0*	15.7*	0.523	0.641	0.267
Speech impairments	35.6*	3.5*	—	4.506	0.412	—
Migraine headaches	35.4*	39.9*	13.3*	0.835	2.089	1.622

Gout, including gouty arthritis	29.3*	74.8*	—	1.356	1.824	—
Asthma	27.5*	4.5*	7.2*	0.958	1.138	0.319
Anemias	26.9*	7.0*	21.7*	1.583	0.389	0.964
Cataracts	26.6*	111.2*	253.3	1.081	1.055	0.986
Hernia of abdominal cavity	26.6*	16.8*	—	0.638	0.213	—
Intervertebral disc disorders	25.5	15.4	12.1	0.729	0.362	0.560
Trouble w/dry (itching) skin, unclassified	24.8*	20.3	7.2*	1.143	0.514	0.330
Paralysis of extremities, complete or partial	22.8*	9.1*	21.7*	3.508	0.469	0.585
Disease of female genital organs	19.9*	—	—	1.171	—	—
Gastritis or duodenitis	19.9*	51.0*	15.7*	0.862	1.074	0.727
Hardening of the arteries	19.4*	64.3*	70.0*	1.037	0.465	1.791
Goiter or other thyroid disorders	19.0*	10.5*	—	0.918	—	—
Frequent constipation	17.1*	30.1*	155.6*	1.118	0.805	0.866
Epilepsy	17.1*	39.9*	—	15.545	6.234	—
Absence of extremities, excluding tip of fingers or toes only	16.2*	58.7*	10.9*	1.174	4.285	0.160
Trouble with ingrown nails	16.2*	49.7*	9.7*	0.466	1.215	0.290
Color blindness	14.2*	4.9*	—	1.069	0.277	—
Emphysema	11.3*	32.2*	12.1*	0.706	0.613	0.660
Glaucoma	10.6*	52.4*	27.7*	0.841	1.514	0.793
Kidney trouble	9.7*	51.7*	30.2*	0.373	2.921	—
Neuralgia or neuritis, unspecified	7.2*	14.0*	—	1.500	1.296	—
Rheumatic fever w/ or w/out heart disease	6.5*	17.5*	—	0.471	1.367	—
Diverticula of intestines	5.2*	8.4*	16.9*	0.280	0.254	0.334
Diseases of prostate	3.8*	12.6*	78.4*	0.409	0.603	2.872

SOURCE: NCHS, 1986a, Table 59, pp. 86-87; — or ——— = no available data.
*Numerators of those quotients with relative standard errors > 30 percent.

Table 4.17 Black Age-Adjusted Cancer Incidence Rates per 100,000, 1974-1983, and Age-Specific Cancer Incidence Rates per 100,000, 1975-1979 and 1980-1984, All Sites Combined, by Sex and Female-to-Male Ratios, United States

Characteristic	Females	Males	Female-to-Male Ratio
Age-Adjusted Rates			
1974	283.4	420.6	0.674
1976	274.6	447.6	0.614
1978	280.6	461.7	0.608
1980	299.5	503.8	0.594
1981	294.4	519.3	0.567
1982	292.2	504.4	0.579
1983	303.6	505.9	0.600
Age-Specific Rates			
1975-1979			
35-44 years	215.3	136.9	1.573
45-54 years	467.2	519.2	0.900
55-64 years	768.8	1,253.6	0.613
65-74 years	1,071.7	2,279.0	0.470
75+ years	1,513.6	3,171.8	0.477
1980-1984			
35-44 years	203.8	132.2	1.542
45-54 years	472.6	545.8	0.866
55-64 years	823.3	1,457.4	0.565
65-74 years	1,203.4	2,589.2	0.465
75+ years	1,635.2	3,498.4	0.655

SOURCE: NCHS, 1986b, and NIH, no date.

rectum. The two highest black male sites were lung and bronchus and prostate gland.

The black female and male five-year annual averages of the age-specific cancer incidence rates for 1975-1979 and 1980-1984 (Table 4.17) show that the risk of cancer among persons 35-44 years of age was much greater for black women than for black men. The average annual percentage of change over time in the male cancer incidence rates by age was insignificant among only the 35- to 44-year-old group. Insignificant changes among females, however, occurred within both the 35- to 44-year-old and the 45- to 54-year-old groups.

The five-year relative survival rates of all sites of cancer among black and white women and men over 35 years of age in NCI's Surveillance, Epidemiology, and End Results (SEER) Program show within each sex-age interval that blacks, as compared to whites, are at greater risk of earlier deaths. As measured by the black-to-white ratios within each sex group, however, there are variations by age in the racial gaps of five-year survivorship: the male gaps are more pronounced among persons under 65 years of age, with the reverse being true thereafter. NCHS (1986b) also shows only slight decreases between 1973-1976 (38%) and 1977-1982 (37%) in the black five-year relative cancer survival rates for all sites of cancer.

Chronic High-Risk Factors

Shifts have occurred among adult blacks throughout this century in their leading causes of death and in the high-risk factors contributing to their early or premature deaths. A major change is reflected in the shift from high-risk factors over which they had relatively little control (e.g., smallpox) to those over which they can exert substantially greater control through behavioral abstinence or behavioral modification. Four fairly common high-risk factors found among middle-aged and aged black populations are cigarette smoking, elevated blood pressure, high serum cholesterol, and obesity.

Cigarette Smoking

The longevity of some heavy smokers far exceeds that of life-long non-smokers, but the risks of early or premature death from certain forms of cancer, as well as from certain heart, cerebrovascular, and respiratory diseases are much greater among smokers than among nonsmokers. For reasons currently unknown, but which may be related to the effectiveness of recent anti-smoking campaigns, the percentages of current smokers among black women and men at age 20-44 years decreased considerably between 1965 and 1985 (Table 4.18). A similar decline among blacks at age 45 or more years is, however, apparent only among black men and not among black women. An encouraging note is that the proportion of former smokers increased between 1965 and 1985 among adult blacks of all ages.

Table 4.18 Percentages of Current and Former Cigarette Smokers Among Blacks, 20-44 and 45 or More Years of Age, in 1965, 1976, 1980, and 1985

Year and Age	Female Smokers		Male Smokers	
	Current	Former	Current	Former
1965				
20-44 years of age	45.0	5.9	67.7	8.3
45+ years of age	20.6	6.0	52.3	17.0
1976				
20-44 years of age	40.1	8.1	57.4	10.2
45+ years of age	28.3	12.4	42.3	30.0
1980				
20-44 years of age	34.3	9.3	47.9	14.2
45+ years of age	25.6	14.1	42.2	26.4
1985				
20-44 years of age	35.5	9.9	40.9	15.8
45+ years of age	26.7	16.9	40.4	32.7

SOURCE: NCHS, 1986b, Table 40, p. 125.

The modal number of cigarettes smoked per day in each of the four years by current female and male smokers in each age group was less than 15. Heavier smoking (i.e., 15+ cigarettes daily) tended to occur more frequently among black males than females. Paradoxically, the growth in reduced smoking among blacks who reported that they smoked fewer than 25 cigarettes daily was also accompanied by a rise between 1965 and 1985 in the proportion of women and men who smoked over 25 cigarettes per day.

Elevated Blood Pressure

The hypertensive prevalence rates of older blacks shown in Table 4.16, based only on respondent assessments, are not sex-specific. The age-adjusted and age-specific rates in Table 4.19, however, are reported separately by sex and are based on medically determined borderline and definite elevated blood pressure. These rates per 100

Table 4.19 Black Age-Adjusted and Age-Specific Rates per 100 Persons, Age 25-74 Years, by Sex and Age, with Medically Determined Borderline or Definite Elevated Blood Pressure, United States, 1960-1962, 1971-1974, and 1976-1980

Rate and Age	Women			Men		
	1960-1962	1971-1974	1976-1980	1960-1962	1971-1974	1976-1980
Borderline						
Age-adjusted						
25-74 years	17.0	17.2	23.9	17.3	20.1	23.1
Age-specific						
25-34 years	7.3	13.5	9.3	10.1	17.5	39.4
35-44 years	13.8	21.7	26.0	16.1	23.7	20.6
45-54 years	20.5	11.6	22.9	21.7	16.3	21.6
55-64 years	32.3	21.1	35.2	25.1	18.0	26.0
65-74 years	13.1*	20.8	34.0	13.5*	29.0	36.6
Definite						
Age-adjusted						
25-74 years	37.7	37.4	26.2	36.3	35.8	29.7
Age-specific						
25-34 years	8.8	10.7	5.8	21.8	16.1	13.4
35-44 years	29.2	28.2	17.4	28.1	36.8	33.2
45-54 years	44.3	49.4	42.9	34.6	37.0	29.3
55-64 years	50.5	54.2	34.2	49.7	49.5	45.7
65-74 years	79.0*	59.8	40.0	63.3*	50.3	32.1

SOURCE: NCHS, 1986b, Tables 44 and 45, pp. 129-130.
* Rates are based on less than 45 persons.

blacks at age 25-74 years in the United States between 1960-1962 and 1976-1980 are also presented by age.

The increases between 1960-1962 and 1976-1980 in the black female and male age-adjusted rates of borderline hypertension are paralleled by decreasing rates of definite hypertension. The patterns of the cross-sectional data do not suggest linear relationships between age and elevated blood pressure, but such relationships may appear in longitudinal data.

One difficulty with the data in Table 4.19, and a difficulty that should be avoided in longitudinal studies of blood pressure levels among blacks, is the failure to differentiate between the subjects with normal blood pressure levels at the time of examination by those who did and did not have a history of elevated blood pressure. In other words, what proportion of the black subjects diagnosed as having normal blood pressure levels were or were not successfully controlling those levels through such behavioral activities as appropriate diets, exercise, or drugs, or any combination thereof?

High-Risk Serum Cholesterol Levels

The age-adjusted and age-specific rates per 100 American blacks at age 25-74 years with medically determined high-risk serum cholesterol levels in 1960-1962, 1971-1974, and 1975-1980 (Table 4.20) reveal some differences by sex and age. These cross-sectional data also show no linear relationships between age and high-risk serum cholesterol levels among adult blacks. The female age-adjusted and age-specific rates generally decreased between the first and last time periods. The reverse pattern occurred among their male counterparts. The male age-specific rates in each age group in 1960-1962 were lower than the corresponding female rates. Among blacks at age 25-44 years in 1976-1980, however, the higher rates were found among men, as opposed to the sexually reversed pattern appearing thereafter in each older age group.

Obesity

The age-adjusted and age-specific rates of blacks medically diagnosed as overweight between 1960-1962 and 1976-1980 (Table 4.21) confirm anew the well-established pattern of greater obesity among

Table 4.20 Black Age-Adjusted and Age-Specific Rates per 100 Persons, Age 25-74 Years, by Sex and Age, with Medically Determined High-risk Serum Cholesterol Levels, United States, 1960-1962, 1971-1974, and 1976-1980

Rate and Age	Women			Men		
	1960-1962	1971-1974	1976-1980	1960-1962	1971-1974	1976-1980
Age-adjusted						
25-74 years	26.8	24.6	22.3	17.1	22.7	23.4
Age-specific						
25-34 years	20.8	19.4	15.6	16.3	22.3	24.8
35-44 years	15.5	14.1	14.3	13.4	23.7	24.5
45-54 years	29.9	27.2	25.8	21.1	20.4	25.3
55-64 years	29.1*	34.4	32.0	13.7	23.0	22.1
65-74 years	50.1*	35.1	29.5	22.9*	25.8	16.6

SOURCE: NCHS, 1986b, Table 46, p. 31.
*Less than 45 persons in the sample.

black women than among black men. Since obesity raises the risk for certain chronic conditions, most alarming is the rising proportion of both overweight women and men within each age-specific group. The only age-specific groups that showed decreased obesity across the years are those of black women at age 35-44 and 55-64 years and of black men at age 25-34 years.

Demographic Differences in Morbidity

Based on the existing literature, the age and sex differences nesting in the reported black-specific rates for acute and chronic conditions (Tables 4.15-4.21) do not appear to be atypical, but, as noted earlier, the relative standard error for much of these data falls far below statistically acceptable standards. The most reliable data include especially cancer incidence and five-year cancer relative survival rates. The black female incidence rates increase with age, whereas their survival rates decrease with age. The black male incidence rates also increase with age, but there is no linear relationship between their age and survival rates.

The age and sex differences among blacks by cigarette smoking can also be supplemented by NLMS data. The proportion smoking was higher among the younger (25-64 years) than older (65+ years) cohort in each sex group. Within-group comparisons of the female and male younger cohorts also showed lower cigarette smoking rates among blacks who were college graduates, married, employed, professionals, and higher earners than among their respective counterparts (U.S. Department of Health and Human Services, 1988, pp. 23-25).

The patterns of sex and age similarities and differences among black female and male cohorts by hypertension, high-risk serum cholesterol level, and obesity did not all remain constant between 1960 and 1980. We do not know the effects of age, period, and cohort on these changing patterns, but some of them point toward better, and others toward poorer, health conditions for some successive sex-age cohorts. For example, the percentage increase between 1960-1962 and 1976-1980 of overweight black men at age 45-54 years from 18.5 to 41.4 was much greater than that of 20.1 to 26.0 among their 55- to 64-year-old counterparts. In addition, in 1960-1962, obesity was slightly higher in the older age group, but, in 1976-1980, it was substantially higher in the younger age group.

Table 4.21 Black Age-Adjusted and Age-Specific Rates per 100 Persons, Age 25-74 Years, by Sex and Age, Medically Designated as Overweight Persons, United States, 1960-1962, 1971-1974, and 1976-1980

Rate and Age	Women			Men		
	1960-1962	1971-1974	1976-1980	1960-1962	1971-1974	1976-1980
Age-adjusted						
25-74 years	47.3	47.8	49.5	24.1	27.6	30.9
Age-specific						
25-34 years	29.6	31.5	33.5	34.3	26.1	17.5
35-44 years	46.1	49.9	40.8	28.6	39.3	40.9
45-54 years	47.8	53.5	61.2	18.5	22.4	41.4
55-64 years	71.4	58.7	59.4	20.1	26.7	26.0
65-74 years	47.8*	49.2	60.8	11.7*	21.6	26.4

SOURCE: NCHS, 1986b, Table 47, p. 132.
*Less than 45 persons in sampled age group.

DISABILITY AND LIMITATION OF ACTIVITY

There are still many gaps in the literature about disabilities and limitations of activities among middle-aged and aged blacks, but the availability of such data has increased enormously during the past few years, owing largely to the enhanced efforts of the Social Security Administration's Division of Disability Studies and NCHS. As may be evident below, there are also considerable differences in the operationalized definitions of disability and limitation of activity and in data-collecting procedures.

Disability

Table 4.22 shows the five-year annual averages between 1980 and 1984 of the number and percentage distributions by age of black female and male disabled-worker claims allowances in the United States. These data, restricted to disabled workers, represent estimates of the population of black yearly worker awards of disability claims "as reflected in the [SSA] administrative records" (U.S. Department of Health and Human Services, 1987, p. 323). SSA defines a disabled worker as a person under 65 years of age who has insured status and who is "unable to engage in any substantial gainful activity, and [has] . . . a disability that can be expected to result in death or to last for a continuous period of not less than 12 months; or be statutorily blind" (U.S. Department of Health and Human Services, 1987, p. 323).

The proportion of blacks among all disabled workers between 1980 and 1984 exceeded their representation in the labor force. A slight majority of black disabled workers lived in the South. The substantially larger number of male than female disabled workers shown in Table 4.22 reflects both the higher employment rates and greater employment in high-risk jobs among males. The modal pre-disability occupations of black women and men respectively were service and structural work. The age distributions of each sex are generally similar, but the median age in the year of entitlement was lower among black males (50.8 years) and females (51.2 years) than among white males (54.0 years) and females (52.9 years).

The five-year annual average between 1980 and 1984 of the mobility of black disabled-worker claims allowance for the two age groups at the time of entitlement of 35-49 years and 50 or more years were

Table 4.22 Five-Year Annual Averages of Number and Percentage Distributions by Age of Black Female and Male Disabled-Worker Claims Allowance, United States, 1980-1984

Age in Year of Entitlement	Black Females	Black Males
Total number	17,256.8	32,555.8
Total percent	100.0	100.0
Under 30 years	8.8	11.7
30-34 years	6.6	7.3
35-39 years	7.4	6.8
40-44 years	8.5	8.1
45-49 years	11.7	10.9
50-54 years	16.9	15.7
55-59 years	21.5	21.4
60+ years	18.6	18.2
Median Age (in years)	51.2	50.8

SOURCE: U.S. Department of Health and Human Services, 1987, pp. 4, 68, 132, 194, and 258.

remarkably similar. About 78 percent of each group were able to go outside with no help, and about 11 percent were able to go outside with help. Less than 6 percent were institutionalized, confined to a general hospital, bedridden, chairbound, or housebound.

The five-year annual average of the number of statutorily blind, disabled workers was significantly higher among black males (599.8) than females (371.0). The proportionate distribution by age among persons over 35 years in each sex group was positively correlated with age. But the percentages of statutorily blind workers in each sex were higher among the 55- to 59-year-olds than among those over 60 years of age (U.S. Department of Health and Human Services, 1987).

Limitation of Activity

Limitation of activity indicates essentially the extent to which persons are functionally dependent on a temporary or permanent basis. Unlike the SSA's disability data, most data about limitation of activity are based on self-reported or respondent-reported assessments. Such NCHS data for older blacks rarely meet the minimum standards of reliability or precision, but the National Health Interview Surveys's practice of oversampling blacks (begun in 1985) has increased somewhat the number of reliable estimates for older blacks.

The national estimates of limitation of activity among civilian, noninstitutionalized blacks (Tables 4.23-4.25) are all based on cross-sectional and respondent-assessed data collected between 1983 and 1985. The degree of activity limitation among older blacks in 1983-1984 (Table 4.23) shows variations by age in each sex group and by sex in each age group. The consistently decreasing male trend of increasing limitation with rising age is not present among the women. The female proportion with no limitation of activity is higher among the 75- to 84-year-olds than among the 65- to 74-year-olds. With the exception of the 75- to 84-year-olds, limited activity is more common among men than among women, a finding also generally true of gender comparisons of the ability to carry on a major activity (e.g., gainful employment).

The available data about limited activity due to chronic conditions among blacks in 1985 (Table 4.24) are not sex-specific, but the age range is much greater than that of Table 4.23. Limited activity is slightly higher among persons over 70 years of age than among the 65- to 69-year-olds. Limited activity in a major activity and in the ability to carry out a major activity is significantly higher among the 65- to 69-year-olds than among their more elderly counterparts.

If we overlook for heuristic purposes the large number of unreliable or imprecise percentages in the data about older blacks who were dependent in performing personal care (Table 4.25) and home management (Table 4.26) activities, the expected rise in dependency with increasing age is present. Gender differences by age are also present. For instance, aged women were generally more dependent in terms of bathing or heavy housework. Among persons over 70 years of age, men were more dependent in terms of preparing meals, shopping, and using the telephone.

Another useful measure of dependency is the rate per 1,000 population of nursing home residents. The national black and white trends between 1973-1974 and 1985 (Table 4.27) by age in these rates are not all coterminous. The black female and male trends in each age group typically showed their significantly greater use of nursing homes in 1985 than in 1973-1974. In contrast, during the same time period there was only a slight increase among white women and a slight decrease among white men.

Table 4.23 Degree of Limitation of Activity Among Blacks, Age 55 or More Years, by Sex and Age, United States, 1983-1984

Sex and Limitation of Activity	Women Age (in years)				Men Age (in years)			
	55-64	65-74	75-84	85+	55-64	65-74	75-84	85+
% No limitation	55.5	49.7	55.0	31.8	61.6	53.9	47.2	40.5*
% Limited, but not in major activity	10.5	16.3	19.6	10.0*	3.5	12.6	11.8	16.2*
% Limited in amount or kind of major activity	19.0	22.0	15.0	32.7	8.4	11.3	26.1	27.0*
% Unable to carry on major activity	14.9	12.0	10.0	24.5	26.5	22.4	14.8	18.9*

SOURCE: NCHS, Havlik et al. (1987, p. 21)
*Statistic does not meet standards of reliability or precision.

Table 4.24 Percentages of Blacks, Age 18 or More Years, with Limitation of Activity Due to Chronic Conditions, by Degree of Limitation and Age, United States, 1985

Limitation of Activity	Age (in years)			
	18-44	45-64	65-69	70+
Number (in thousands)	11,889	4,432	818	1,441
% With no limitation of activity	91.1	69.3	49.5	51.6
% With limitation of activity	8.9	30.7	50.5	48.4
% with limitation in major activity	6.9	25.2	39.4	29.1
% unable to carry on major activity	3.5	15.3	28.2	12.1
% limited in amount or kind of major activity	3.4	9.9	11.1	17.0
% limited, but not in major activity	2.0	5.6	11.1	19.4

SOURCE: NCHS (1986a, Table 68, p. 108).

Table 4.25 Percentages of Blacks, Age 55 or More Years, Dependent in Performing Personal Care Activities, by Sex and Age, National Health Interview Survey, 1984

Sex and Activity	Age (in years)				
	55-59	60-64	65-74	75-84	85+
Women					
% Bathing	7.0*	3.7*	4.4*	12.2	34.5*
% Dressing	4.9*	0.8*	4.0*	6.9*	19.9*
% Using the toilet	3.1*	—	2.2*	6.9*	25.8*
% Getting in and out of beds/chairs	4.0*	1.3*	2.8*	5.8*	15.4*
% Eating	—	—	1.4*	0.8*	4.6*
Men					
% Bathing	2.6*	2.0*	4.4*	6.2	27.0*
% Dressing	1.1*	1.1*	3.2*	12.5	30.6*
% Using the toilet	—	0.9*	1.7*	4.8	5.1*
% Getting in and out of beds/chairs	1.1*	0.9*	1.4*	1.4*	5.1*
% Eating	—	1.1*	0.4*	2.3*	5.1*

SOURCE: NCHS (1988).
*The rate per 1,000 persons from the 1984 National Health Survey falls below the standards of reliability or precision.

Table 4.26 Estimated Percentages of Blacks, Age 65 or More Years of Age, Dependent in Performing Home Management Activities, by Sex and Age, National Health Interview Survey

Activity	Women Age (in years)				Men Age (in years)			
	65+	65-74	75-84	85+	65+	65-74	75-84	85+
Preparing meals	6.4	3.1*	9.5*	20.8*	6.5	2.5*	9.6*	41.6*
Shopping	12.4	5.7	20.4	34.9*	8.5	4.6	11.6*	41.6*
Managing money	5.7	2.1*	8.3*	25.4*	6.0	4.0*	7.5*	24.4*
Using telephone	2.8*	2.1*	3.5	5.8*	2.0*	0.7*	2.6*	14.4
Light housework	7.5	4.2*	11.1	20.8*	7.0	3.9*	10.0*	31.5
Heavy housework	27.3	19.2	37.6	51.6*	14.2	9.5	19.0	46.3

SOURCE: NCHS (1988a).
*Percentage does not meet standards of reliability or precision.

Table 4.27 Black and White Nursing Home Resident Rates by Sex and Age, United States, 1973-1974, 1977, and 1985, and 1985-to-1973-1974 Ratios

Race and Year	Females Age (in years)					Males Age (in years)				
	Under 65	65+	65-74	75-84	85+	Under 65	65+	65-74	75-84	85+
Black										
1973-1974	0.5	24.8	11.0	31.8	113.5	0.6	18.1	11.2	19.4	92.0
1977	0.8	36.1	17.9	40.5	158.1	0.9	23.0	17.2	22.9	86.7
1985	0.6	39.4	16.0	45.1	162.7	1.1	28.5	14.5	45.6	95.6
White										
1973-1974	0.7	57.8	13.4	71.9	310.0	0.6	31.2	11.3	41.6	192.3
1977	1.0	60.9	15.7	78.7	217.1	0.8	31.1	12.1	47.1	152.9
1985	0.8	60.2	13.7	68.5	259.2	0.8	29.2	10.5	43.0	150.8
1985-to-1973-1974 ratio										
Black	1.200	1.589	1.454	1.418	1.434	1.833	1.575	1.295	2.351	1.039
White	1.143	1.042	1.022	0.952	0.836	1.333	0.936	0.929	1.034	0.784

SOURCE: NCHS, (1988b). These rates exclude residents in personal care or domiciliary care homes. All Hispanics were classified as white in 1973-1974 and 1977.

Racial and gender ratios of rates of nursing home residents in the United States in 1973-1974, 1977, and 1985 provide a comparative perspective on an early and still pervasive issue in ethnogerontology, viz., racial parity in nursing homes (see, e.g., Jackson, 1973b, 1976). A comparison of percentage changes between 1973-1974 and 1985 in each black-to-white female age group specified in Table 4.27 showed narrowing gaps. Gaps in the corresponding black-to-white male groups widened among those less than age 65 years and 65-74 years. The black female-to-male ratios narrowed only among persons under age 75 years. The white female-to-male ratios widened only among the 65- to 74-year-olds. Thus, there were some racial similarities and differences.

Most striking are the higher black than white rates among both the 65- to 74-year-old women and men in 1977 and 1985. This cohort (all born between 1910 and 1919) had higher white than black birth rates, but lower white than black infant mortality rates of their offspring. Spousal presence in this age group in 1983-1984 was also more common among whites. Other data suggest that living alone and limitation of activity were also more common among these blacks than among their white counterparts. These variables help explain this greater black than white nursing home resident rate (see Kovar, 1988).

Demographic Differences in Disability and Limitation of Activities

The limited data on disabled-worker claims allowance show substantially higher male (65.4%) than female (34.6%) claims allowance, as well as consistent increases with age under 65 years. The lack of substantial age differences by mobility also seems to be real rather than apparent, owing mostly, if not entirely, to the specialized population of this data set.

Sex and age differences among older blacks by limitation of activity, dependency, and nursing home residency are much greater than are those among worker-claim allowance recipients. Kovar and LaCroix (1987, p. 1) suggest "that data based solely on working populations are not sufficient for investigating age-related changes in the proportion of people with difficulty or inability to perform a specified task." We quite agree, but stress especially the fact that much of the available NCHS data about limitation of activities and dependency among older blacks still fall far below the acceptable standards of reliability, or, worse, are simply missing, owing to insufficient sampling size. Consequently, for example, we could not determine the age differences between the two cohorts of black women at age 55-59 years and 60-64 years by their dependency in performing personal care activities.

The generally higher rate of nursing home residents between 1973-1974 and 1985 among aged black and white women than among aged black and white men cannot be explained adequately by the available cross-sectional data. But, as Kovar (1986) essentially suggested, the traditional explanation of simply greater living alone among aged women than men may be invalid. Instead, the higher risks of dying or of institutionalization among aged persons living alone occur among those "who did not have children or siblings, frequent social contact, recent medical care, or high self-perception of their health" (Kovar, 1986, p. 5). Almost one-half of all aged blacks in households live in nonfamilial households, most of whom live alone, and the vast majority of aged blacks are not in nursing homes. Therefore, although Kovar (1986) reported no race-specific data, a reasonable hypothesis is that her findings also apply to aged blacks.

RESPONDENT-ASSESSED AND SELF-REPORTED HEALTH STATUSES

The health statuses of middle-aged and aged blacks reported in the aging and related literature are almost always subjectively measured by respondent assessments or self-reports. Clinical determinations of those health statuses are still too rare. While self-reports cannot replace clinical diagnoses, Shanas and Maddox (1985) believe that they do contain useful and reliable data. That judgment, however, is based on a longitudinal study of mostly white elderly community volunteers who received periodic reports of their clinical examinations. To the best of our knowledge, no study has yet used a representative sample of middle-aged or aged blacks in order to determine cross-sectionally or longitudinally the relationships existing between or among their respondent-assessed, self-reported, and clinically determined health statuses. Until such studies are forthcoming, we are forced to rely mostly on respondent assessments and self-reports.

Respondent Assessments

Using chi-square, the respondent-assessed health status of older blacks in the United States in 1983-84 (Table 4.28) shows no statistically significant differences among the age groups within each sex or between the sexes within each age group.

Also based on chi-square, the respondent-assessed health statuses of adult blacks and whites in the United States in 1985 (Table 4.29) were not statistically significant by race among persons at age 25-44 years or 65 or more years. Among persons at age 45-64 years, however, the white respondent-assessed health statuses were significantly better. For example, fair or poor health status was reported for 33.1 percent of these blacks and only 16.9 percent of these whites.

Self-Reports

The above finding of racially insignificant differences among the aged by respondent-assessed health status corresponds well to similar findings by clinically determined health status (see, e.g., Nowlin, 1977, 1979; Ostfeld et al., 1971), but not with self-reported health status (see, e.g., Ferron, 1981; NCHS, 1986a; and Shanas, 1977). Self-reported health data usually show substantially greater judgments of fair or poor health statuses among blacks.

While the factors explaining this real or apparent racial difference are not yet known, Krause (1987, p. 74) reported its persistence even after controlling "for the effects of stress, response bias, age, sex, marital status, education, and depressive symptoms." Had he also controlled his 1984 random sample of community black and white elderly in Galveston, Texas, by such factors as major lifetime occupation, all sources and amounts of an individual's total money income during the year preceding the interview, living arrangements, and number of rooms per person in a household, his finding might have been different. That is, we are not yet convinced that comparable elderly blacks and whites differ significantly by their self-reported health statuses.

Demographic Differences About Subjective Health Status

The ethnogerontologic and related literature about subjective health status of older blacks focuses most heavily on black and white comparisons. The commonplace finding by self-reports (see, e.g., Krause, 1987), but not always by respondent assessments, is subjectively poorer health among blacks. The most recent cross-sectional data show insignificant relationships between sex or age and subjective health

Table 4.28 Respondent-Assessed Health Status of Blacks, Age 55 or More Years, by Sex and Age, United States, 1983-1984

Health Status	Women Age (in years)				Men Age (in years)			
	55-64	65-74	75-84	85+	55-64	65-74	75-84	85+
% Excellent or Very Good	24.3	23.8	25.4	21.8*	30.8	26.2	27.7	24.3*
% Good	27.0	20.6	21.6	25.5	27.3	26.0	23.1	24.3
% Fair or Poor	47.6	54.5	50.8	50.0	41.4	47.4	48.1	48.6

SOURCE: NCHS, Havlik et al. (1987) p. 21.
*Statistic does not meet the standards of reliability or precision.

Table 4.29 Black and White Respondent-Assessed Health Statuses, Age 25 or More Years, by Age, United States, 1985

Health Status	Women Age (in years)			Men Age (in years)		
	25-44	*45-64*	*65+*	*25-44*	*45-64*	*65+*
% Excellent	29.9	15.1	8.3	44.0	28.3	16.6
% Very Good	26.8	18.8	16.8	30.9	26.0	20.5
% Good	30.1	32.9	27.8	19.7	28.7	33.0
% Fair	10.3	21.6	28.3	4.2	11.3	20.9
% Poor	2.8	11.5	18.8	1.2	5.6	9.1

SOURCE: NCHS, (1986a).

status among older blacks. This leads us to speculate that the impact of age on the subjective health statuses of older blacks is negligible.

SUMMARY AND CONCLUSIONS

The comparative data presented herein about the aggregated demographic and physical health conditions of middle-aged and aged blacks in the United States, coupled with Jackson's (1967, 1973a, 1981, 1985) previous reviews of the related literature, provide no valid and reliable findings about age changes in "the blacklands of gerontology." But they do contain much fruitful information—some old, some new— about both similarities and differences among these blacks by sex, age, and marital status, and, to a far lesser extent, by race, geographical location, household size, income, education, and employment.

The fundamental task of identifying and verifying age changes in the physical and mental health conditions of older blacks has been hampered severely in the past by the extreme paucity of causally-oriented sequential cross-sectional studies on the macrolevel and longitudinal studies on the microlevel of representative samples of black birth cohorts. Yet, even if such studies were already available or in progress, there is still the critical problem of isolating age changes from period and cohort changes (see Maddox & Campbell, 1985), as well as the highly reasonable proposition that there are generally no systematic, systemic, and inevitable age changes in the physical health conditions of adult blacks in the United States.

The propitious growth during the past few years in the availability of national data about health conditions and their determinants from sequential cross-sectional and longitudinal investigations using adult black subjects has clearly helped to reduce some of the most glaring gaps in our knowledge about and understanding of these blacks and, to a lesser extent, the populations they represent.

Although the various volumes of the Report of the Secretary's Task Force on Black and Minority Health (U.S. Department of Health and Human Services, 1985-1986) contained no novel data or research recommendations and failed to codify adequately the then existing research data and findings about the physical, dental, and mental health of adult blacks in the United States, and especially so of the American natives among them, they may well have prompted increased federal research interest about blacks, or, at the very least, encouraged the continuation of such ongoing research interests supported by federal funding.

NCHS, followed by NCI, seems to have taken the lead among federal agencies that fund internal or external research in increasing our knowledge and understanding of black health conditions and their sociodemographic and other relevant variations. This leading role is, perhaps, exemplified best by the oversampling of blacks since 1985 in the annual National Health Interview Survey. Even so, however, this black oversampling does not resolve problems of missing or unreliable data. Sampling data about the health conditions of living blacks are far more reliable when the population is black as opposed to that of all races.

Drury and Powell's (1987) report on the estimated black prevalence rate of known diabetes mellitus illustrates well NCHS's increasing focus on intra-black differences, such as those between insulin dependents and noninsulin dependents, and explanations of black and white differences. Finding that age, sex, education, marital status, living arrangement, family income, geographical location of residence, and geographic region did not appear to explain the racially different prevalence rates, Drury and Powell (1987, p. 7) suspected that obesity might be an explanatory variable since "persistent obesity is a major risk factor" for noninsulin dependent diabetes and obesity is much higher among blacks.

Aware, however, of the lack of "historically-comparable, replicated measures of the prevalence of diagnosed and undiagnosed diabetes" among blacks in the past, Drury and Powell (1987) pointed out that the first estimates of diagnosed and undiagnosed diabetes available for a national probability sample of American adults that included black subjects came from the second National Health and Nutrition Examination Survey (NHANES II), 1976-1980, and that comparable data should be forthcoming from NHANES III, 1988-1993. In light as well of the limited studies on the etiology of noninsulin-dependent diabetes among blacks and changes since 1963 in their prevalence rates of known diabetes, they emphasize current research needs for good studies about black risks of becoming diabetic, factors affecting their rising prevalence rates (e.g., better identification of new cases, increased survivorship, or changes in the ratio of diagnosed to undiagnosed diabetes), and the applicability of explanations of changing diabetic prevalence rates among whites to blacks. Their research suggestions constitute a useful paradigm for investigations of other major diseases among blacks.

The preliminary reports of the NCHS 1984 cross-sectional Supplement on Aging about persons at age 55 years and over contain useful findings and hypotheses about such topics as contacts with family, friends, and neighbors among persons living alone (Kovar, 1986), ability to perform work-related activities (Kovar & LaCroix, 1987), functional limitations (Dawson, Hendershot, & Fulton, 1987), prevalence and impact of urinary problems (Harris, 1986), impaired senses for sound and light (Havlik, 1986), and use of community services (Stone, 1986).

These reports contain no black-specific data and the black samples are extremely small. But the findings and hypotheses probably apply about equally as well to middle-aged and aged blacks as to comparable whites. One example is Stone's (1986, p. 3) commonsensical speculation "that despite their limitations, moderately to severely limited elderly persons living alone were more likely to participate in senior center programs for social support. In contrast, those living with others were perhaps not as likely to use senior centers because they received this support at home."

At the very least, representative and sufficiently large samples of the populations of middle-aged and aged blacks could be used to test the hypotheses nesting within these NCHS preliminary and subsequent reports. New studies using older black samples to test these hypotheses could also try to distinguish between moderately to severely limited elderly persons living alone who do and do not participate in senior center programs for social support. Similar distinctions between their counterparts who do not live alone would also be useful.

What is most exciting about the 1984 Supplement on Aging is that it is the basis for the Longitudinal Study on Aging, a collaborative project between NCHS and the National Institute of Aging "that involves matches with existing records, such as death certificates, for all of the people in the Supplement on Aging, and reinterviews with samples of people who were in the 1984 study" (Kovar, 1988, p. 1). Reinterviews in 1986 with a sample of persons who were over 70 years of age and not institutionalized in 1984 showed that most of the respondents still had the same living arrangements, a higher proportion of nursing home residents among persons who lived alone than among those not living alone in 1984, and that age and functional status in 1984 were the two most powerful factors associated with nursing home residency in 1986 (Kovar, 1988, p. 2). Although Kovar (1988) did not report any black-specific data in this preliminary report, her findings and further research suggestions also seem to apply to blacks.

Consequently, one of our three most important research suggestions about the causal relationships among health conditions, age, and aging among American blacks is to encourage the further creation of relevant data sets and more use of secondary data sets, such as the Longitudinal Study of Aging and the SSA's ten-year Retirement History Study (1969-1979). Maddox and Campbell (1985, pp. 23-28) provide a brief, but good general discussion of emerging data bases and longitudinal studies.

Gibson and Jackson's (1987) excellent analysis of relationships between elderly black health, physical functioning, and informal support, based on the national probability sample of the Three-Generation Black Family Study raises or raises anew extremely useful research issues. These issues include more precise identification of "the contrasting social, psychological, and informal support characteristics of" black functional health subgroups, determination of the linear and nonlinear relationships between age and health conditions, modifications of informal social networks and support among successive black elderly cohorts, relationships between the amount of emotional support and physical functioning, and, in line with Jackson's (1973a) and Drury and Powell's (1987) suggestions, better identification and explanation of the similarities and differences between black and white health conditions.

Gibson and Jackson (1987, p. 446) indicated that "research on the black old should be conducted within a framework of their lifetime experiences and major social change, overlaying differential experiences within subgroups of the black old and across cultures." We recommend using their three-tiered framework for future research about the health conditions of all adult blacks. In fact, they hope that the issues they raised "will stimulate thought and provide an initial framework for future research on the interplay of . . . [health, functioning, and informal supports] and the health care needs of black adults as they age in American society" (Gibson & Jackson, 1987, p. 448). Sharing that hope, our second major recommendation is the testing by ethnogerontologists of the Gibson-Jackson theoretical framework.

Our third recommendation is a longstanding one, specifically on the misuse of the variable of race in most epidemiological, gerontological, and related studies (see especially Caplan, Robinson, French, Caldwell, & Shinn, 1976; Cooper, 1984; Gibson & Jackson, 1987; Jackson, 1967, 1980, 1985, 1988). A glaring example of the misuse of race seems to appear in Pfeiffer's (1975, pp. 433-434) ten-item Short Portable Mental Status Questionnaire (SPMSQ), which was designed "to determine the presence and degree of intellectual impairment" among elderly persons. The test score (0-10) and intellectual functioning are inversely related, so that the higher the score, the greater the degree of intellectual impairment. The scoring instructions call for allowing "one more error if subject has only a grade school education," "one less error if subject has had education beyond high school," and *"one more error for black subjects,* using identical education criteria" (Pfeiffer, 1975, p. 441). Pfeiffer's (1975, p. 441) justification for those instructions is that, "The data suggest that both education and race influence performance on the Mental Status Questionnaire and they must accordingly be taken into account in evaluating the score attained by an individual."

Given the relatively widespread use of SPMSQ by health and social service agencies for the elderly, this misuse of race is particularly disturbing in that some blacks with moderate or severe organic impairment may be misdiagnosed and fall below the minimum score required for receipt of services. Moreover, the rising educational level of the elderly may also necessitate some modification of the educational scoring.

In addition, the scoring instruction for item 9 on the SPMSQ, "What was your mother's maiden name?" in "Question 9 does not need to be verified. It is scored correct if a female first name plus a last name other than subject's last name is given" (Pfeiffer, 1975, p. 441). When Mary Brown, born to Susie and Timothy Brown, marries Willie Brown, what is Mary Brown's maiden name? Brown, of course! When Ruby Goldburg, an unwed mother, names her infant son Rubin Goldburg, and years later the son's response to item 9 is Goldburg, why is his response incorrect? In short, this question or its scoring system does not reflect sociocultural reality or diversity.

A methodological problem much related to the misuse of race is the continuing need to disentangle race, social class, and socioeconomic status. Cooper's (1984) view that black and white socioeconomic statuses are not directly comparable, and Campbell and Parker's (1983) rejection of the Duncan Socioeconomic Index as a measure of socioeconomic status should be considered in developing new measures for black and white comparisons of health conditions. New measures of social class and socioeconomic status among blacks are also needed for intra-black comparisons of health conditions.

Finally, we are concerned about researchers who use the concept of *excess*, as in excess deaths, in comparing black and white health conditions, and then use those comparisons in a valuative sense or as the basis for proposing public policies. For example, a task force on black and minority health used the "technique of excess deaths . . . [as] an appropriate tool for setting priorities relevant to policy formation" (U.S. Department of Health and Human Services, 1985-1986, p. 18). Following Rothman's (1987) suggestion, our comparisons of middle-aged and aged blacks and whites were "made only to learn about the differences, and not to suggest any policy or set of values." Racially comparative studies of adult health conditions in the United States also need to place much greater priority on learning about and explaining the differences than on using white health conditions as the explicit or implicit standard for black health conditions.

REFERENCES

Campbell, R., & Parker, R. N. (1983). Substantive and statistical considerations in the interpretation of multiple measures of SES. *Social Forces, 62,* 450-466.

Caplan, R. D., Robinson, E. A. R., French, J. R. P., Jr., Caldwell, J. R., & Shinn, M. (1976). *Adhering to medical regimens: Pilot experiments in patient education and social support.* Ann Arbor: Institute for Social Research, The University of Michigan.

Centers for Disease Control. (1987). Public use tape of AIDS victims.

Christensen, B. J. (1988). The costly retreat from marriage. *The Public Interest, 91* (Spring), 59-66.

Cooper, R. (1984). A note on the biologic concept of race and its application in epidemiologic research. *American Heart Journal, 108,* 715-723.

Dawson, D., Hendershot, G., & Fulton, J. (1987). Aging in the eighties: Functional limitations of individuals age 65 years and over. *Advance data from vital and health statistics.* (No. 133. DHHS Pub. No. [PHS] 87-1250). Hyattsville, MD: Public Health Service.

Drury, T. F., & Powell, A. L. (1987). Prevalence of known diabetes among black Americans. *Advance data from vital and health statistics.* (No. 130, DHHS Pub. No. [PHS] 87-1250). Hyattsville, MD: Public Health Service.

Ferron, D. T. (compiler). (1981). *Disability survey 72, Disabled and nondisabled adults, a monograph.* (Research Report No. 56, SSA Publication No. 13-11812). Washington, DC: U.S. Government Printing Office.

Friedman, S. R., Sotheran, J. L., Abdul-Quader, A., Primm, B. J., Des Jarlais, D. C., Kleinman, P., Mauge, C., Goldsmith, D. S., El-Sadr, W., & Maslansky, R. (1987). The AIDS epidemic among blacks and Hispanics. *The Milbank Quarterly, 65* (Suppl. 2), 455-467.

Fumenton, M. A. (1987). AIDS: Are heterosexuals at risk? *Commentary, 84,* 21-27.

Gibson, R. C., & Jackson, J. S. (1987). The health, physical functioning, and informal supports of the black elderly. *The Milbank Quarterly, 65* (Suppl. 2), 421-454.

Harris, T. (1986). Aging in the eighties. Prevalence and impact of urinary problems in individuals age 65 years and over. *Preliminary data from the Supplement on Aging to the National Health Interview Survey, United States, January-June 1984. Advance data from vital and health statistics.* (No. 121. DHHS Pub. No. [PHS] 86-1250). Hyattsville, MD: Public Health Service.

Havlik, R. J. (1986). Aging in the eighties: Impaired senses for sound and light in persons age 65 years and over. *Preliminary data from the Supplement on Aging to the National Health Interview Survey, United States, January-June 1984. Advance data from vital and health statistics.* (No. 125. DHHS Pub. No. [PHS] 86-1250. Hyattsville, MD: Public Health Service.

Jackson, J. J. (1967). Social gerontology and the Negro: A review. *The Gerontologist, 7,* 168-178.

Jackson, J. J. (1973a). The blacklands of gerontology. In V. M. Brantly & M. R. Brown (Eds.), *Readings in gerontology,* (pp. 78-97). St. Louis: C. V. Mosby. (Reprinted from *Aging and Human Development,* 1971, *2,* 156-171)

Jackson, J. J. (1973b). Black women in a racist society. In C. Willie, B. Kramer, & B. Brown (Eds.), *Racism and mental health* (pp. 185-268). Pittsburgh: University of Pittsburgh Press.

Jackson, J. J. (1976) The plight of older black women in the United States. *The Black Scholar, 7,* 47-55.

Jackson, J. J. (1980). *Minorities and aging.* Belmont, CA: Wadsworth.

Jackson, J. J. (1981). Urban black Americans. In A. Harwood (Ed.), *Ethnicity and medical care* (pp. 37-129). Cambridge, MA: Harvard University Press.

Jackson, J. J. (1985). Race, national origin, ethnicity, and aging. In R. H. Binstock & E. Shanas (Eds.), *Handbook of aging and the social sciences* (2nd Ed.) (pp. 264-303). New York: Van Nostrand Reinhold.

Jackson, J. J. (1987). *Aging black women and public policies.* Keynote address, Conference on Aging Black Women, Oakland, CA (in modified copy in *The Black Scholar, 19,* 31-43, 1988).

Jackson, J. J. (1988). Social determinants of the health of aging black populations in the United States. In J. S. Jackson (Ed.), *The black American elderly: Research on physical and psychosocial health.* New York: Springer.

Jackson, J. J., & Perry, C. (1988). Trends in the black and white crossovers in age-specific death rates and probabilities of dying, United States, 1966-1984. *Journal of Minority Aging, 13,* 1-17.

Kitagawa, E. M., & Hauser, P. M. (1973). *Differential mortality in the United States: A study in socioeconomic epidemiology.* Cambridge, MA: Harvard University Press.

Kovar, M. G. (1986). Aging in the eighties, age 65 years and over and living alone: Contacts with family, friends, and neighbors. *Preliminary data from the Supplement on*

Aging to the National Health Interview Survey: United States, January-June 1984. Advance data from vital and health statistics. (No. 116. DHHS Pub. No. [PHS] 86-1250). Hyattsville, MD: Public Health Service.

Kovar, M. G. (1988). Aging in the Eighties: People living alone—two years later. *Advance data from vital and health statistics.* (No. 149. DHHS Pub. No. [PHS] 86-1250). Hyattsville, MD: Public Health Center.

Kovar, M. G., & LaCroix, A. Z. (1987). Aging in the eighties, Ability to perform work-related activities. *Advance data from the Supplement on Aging to the National Health Interview Survey, United States, 1984. Advance data from vital and health statistics.* (No. 136. DHHS Pub. No. [PHS] 87-1250). Hyattsville, MD: Public Health Service.

Krause, N. (1987). Stress in racial differences in self-reported health among the elderly. *The Gerontologist, 27,* 72-76.

Maddox, G. L., & Campbell, R. T. (1985). Scope, concepts, and methods in the study of aging. In R. H. Binstock & E. Shanas (Eds.), *Handbook of aging and the social sciences* (2nd Ed.) (pp. 3-31). New York: Van Nostrand Reinhold.

Mergenhagen, P. M., Lee, B. A., & Gove, W. R. (1985). Till death do us part: Recent changes in the relationship between marital status and mortality. *Social Science Research, 70(1),* 53-56.

Mott, F. L., & Haurin, R. J. (1985). Factors affecting mortality in the years surrounding retirement. In H. S. Parnes, J. E. Crowley, R. J. Haurin, L. J. Less, W. R. Morgan, F. L. Mott, & G. Nestel (Eds.), *Retirement among American men* (pp. 31-56). Lexington, MA: Lexington Books and D. C. Heath.

National Cancer Institute. (no date). *Cancer among blacks and other minorities: Statistical profiles.* (NIH Publication No. 86-2785). Bethesda, MD: National Institute of Health.

National Center for Health Statistics. (1972, 1974, 1982-1987). *Vital statistics of the United States. Vol. II. Mortality, Part A. Public Health Service.* Washington, DC: U.S. Government Printing Office.

National Center for Health Statistics. (1986a). *Current estimates from the National Health Interview Survey, United States, 1985. Vital and health statistics.* (Series 10. No. 160. DHHS Pub. No. [PHS] 86-1588). Washington, DC: U.S. Government Printing Office.

National Center for Health Statistics. (1986b). *Health, United States, 1986.* (DHHS Pub. No. [PHS] 87-1232). Public Health Service. Washington, DC: U.S. Government Printing Office.

National Center for Health Statistics. (1987). *Health statistics on older persons, United States, 1986. Vital and health statistics.* (Series 3, No. 25. DHHS Pub. No. [PHS] 87-1409). Public Health Service. Washington, DC: U.S. Government Printing Office.

National Center for Health Statistics. (1988a, 1988b). Printouts of table materials forwarded by request prior to publication.

Nowlin, J. B. (1977). Successful aging: Health and social factors in an interracial population. *Black Aging, 2,* 10-17.

Nowlin, J. B. (1979). Geriatric health status: Influence of race and economic status. *Journal of Minority Aging, 4,* 93-98.

Ortmeyer, C. E. (1974). Variations in mortality, morbidity, and health care by marital status. In C. I. Erhart & J. C. Berlin (Eds.), *Mortality and morbidity in the United States* (pp. 159-188). Cambridge, MA: Harvard University Press.

Ostfeld, A. M., Shekelle, R. B., Tufo, H. M., Wieland, A. M., Kilbridge, J. A., Drori, J., & Klawans, H. (1971). Cardiovascular disease in an elderly poor urban population. *American Journal of Public Health, 61*, 19-29.

Pfeiffer, E. (1975). A short portable mental status questionnaire for the assessment of organic brain deficit in elderly patients. *Journal of the American Geriatrics Society, 23*, 433-441.

Reid, J. D., Lee, E. S., Jedlicka, D., & Shin, Y. (1977). Trends in black health. *Phylon, 38*, 105-116.

Rothman, K. J. (1987). Personal communication to J. J. Jackson.

Shanas, E. (1977). *National survey of the aged, final report.* (Grant No. #57823). Baltimore, MD: Office of Research and Statistics, Social Security Administration.

Shanas, E., & Maddox, G. L. (1985). Health, health resources, and the utilization of care. In R. H. Binstock & E. Shanas (Eds.), *Handbook of aging and the social sciences* (pp. 697-726). New York: Van Nostrand Reinhold.

Stone, R. (1986). Aging in the eighties, age 65 years and over—use of community services. *Preliminary data from the Supplement on Aging to the National Health Interview Survey: United States, January-June 1985, Advance data from vital and health statistics.* (No. 124. DHHS Pub. No. [PHS] 86-1250). Hyattsville, MD: Public Health Service.

U.S. Bureau of the Census. (1980-1983, 1984d, and 1985a). *Marital status and living arrangements for March 1979-March 1984.* (Current Population Reports, Series P-20). Washington, DC: U.S. Government Printing Office.

U.S. Bureau of the Census. (1984a). *Educational attainment in the United States: March 1981 and 1980.* (Current Population Reports, Series P-20, No. 390). Washington, DC: U.S. Government Printing Office.

U.S. Bureau of the Census. (1984b). *General housing characteristics for the United States and regions: 1983, Annual housing survey:1983, Part A.* (Current Housing Reports, Series 83). Washington, DC: U.S. Government Printing Office.

U.S. Bureau of the Census. (1984c). *Money income of households, families, and persons in the United States: 1982.* (Current Population Reports, Series P-60, No. 142). Washington, DC: U. S. Government Printing Office.

U.S. Bureau of the Census. (1985b). *Household and family characteristics: March 1984.* (Current Population Reports, Series P-20, No. 398). Washington, DC: U.S. Government Printing Office.

U.S. Bureau of the Census. (1987a). *Estimates of the population of the United States, by age, sex, and race: 1980-1986.* (Current Population Reports, Series P-25). Washington, DC: U.S. Government Printing Office.

U.S. Bureau of the Census. (1987b). *Educational attainment in the United States: March 1982 to 1985.* (Current Population Reports). Washington, DC: U.S. Government Printing Office.

U.S. Bureau of the Census. (1987c). *Money income of households, families, and persons in the United States: 1985.* (Current Population Reports, Series P-60, No. 156). Washington, DC: U.S. Government Printing Office.

U.S. Bureau of the Census. (1987d). *Poverty in the United States: 1985.* (Current Population Reports, Series P-60, No. 158). Washington DC: U.S. Government Printing Office.

U.S. Bureau of the Census. (1987e). *Household and family characteristics: March 1986.* (Current Population Reports, Series P-20, No. 419). Washington, DC: U.S. Government Printing Office.

U.S. Bureau of the Census. (1988). *Educational attainment in the United States: March 1987 and (1986).* (Current Population Reports, Series P-20, No. 428). Washington, DC: U.S. Government Printing Office.

U.S. Department of Health and Human Services. (No date). *1986 annual cancer statistics review.* (NIH Publication No. 87-2789). Division of Cancer Prevention and Control Surveillance Operations Research Branch.

U.S. Department of Health and Human Services. (1985-1986). *Report of the secretary's task force on black and minority health,* (Vols. I-VII). Washington, DC: U.S. Department of Health and Human Services.

U.S. Department of Health and Human Services. (1987). *Characteristics of Social Security disability insurance beneficiaries.* (SSA Pub. No. 13-11947). Washington, DC: U.S. Government Printing Office.

U.S. Department of Health and Human Services. (1988). *First data book, A mortality study of one million persons by demographic, social, and economic factors: 1979-1981 follow-up, U.S. National Longitudinal Mortality Study.* (NIH Publication No. 88-2896). Bethesda, MD: National Institutes of Health.

U.S. Department of Labor, Bureau of Labor Statistics. (1985). *Handbook of labor statistics.* (Bulletin 2217). Washington, DC: U.S. Government Printing Office.

U.S. Department of Labor, Bureau of Labor Statistics. (1986). *Employment and earnings.* Washington, DC: U.S. Government Printing Office.

CHAPTER 5

Aging and Health Among Southwestern Hispanics

KYRIAKOS S. MARKIDES
JEANNINE COREIL
LINDA PERKOWSKI ROGERS

INTRODUCTION

Hispanics constitute the second largest ethnic minority population in the United States, approaching 20 million people. It is also a rapidly growing population that should overtake the black population in numbers before the end of the century. Despite its size and importance, Hispanics remain somewhat mysterious and poorly understood.

Most Hispanics live in the five southwestern states where they are mostly Mexican Americans. Demographically speaking, Mexican Americans are a young population primarily because of high fertility and a continuous flow of immigrants who tend to be younger. However, like other groups the Mexican American population is aging, with the number of the elderly rising.

Although there has been a long tradition of research on the health care behavior of Mexican Americans (Andersen, 1981; Hoppe &

AUTHORS' NOTE: Parts of Chapter 5 were previously published and are used in substantially revised form with permission from the publisher. The original manuscript was: Markides, K. S., & Coreil, J. (1988). "The health status of Hispanic elderly in the Southwest." In S. R. Applewhite (Ed.), *Hispanic elderly in transition* (pp. 35-59). Westport, CT: Greenwood Press. Copyright © 1988 by Steven R. Applewhite. Revised and reprinted with permission.

Heller, 1975; Madsen, 1964; Rubel, 1966; Saunders, 1954; Weaver, 1973), much less interest has been shown in understanding the health status of this population (Markides & Coreil, 1986). Among factors accounting for this have been the lack of adequate data and definitional problems of what constitutes a "Mexican American" or "Hispanic." Yet research on the health of Mexican Americans and other Hispanics is increasing, and the recently completed Hispanic Health and Nutrition Examination Survey is likely to generate highly useful knowledge on the health and health care behavior of this population.

This chapter aims at providing an overview of the evidence on the current health status of Southwestern Hispanics with particular focus on middle-aged and older persons. We begin with an account of the general mortality situation in 1970 and 1980, followed by the evidence on cardiovascular diseases, cancer, diabetes, and other diseases. Finally, we review data on functional health indicators derived from survey data.

GENERAL MORTALITY

Ellis's work with 1949-1951 data from San Antonio and Houston (Ellis, 1959, 1962) demonstrated that Spanish-surname whites had higher mortality rates and lower life expectancy than did Anglos (other whites), and this was particularly so for women (see Roberts, 1977, for more discussion). Roberts and Askew (1972), analyzing 1949-1951 data from Houston, found that the mortality situation of Mexican Americans at that time was even less favorable than that of blacks. However, their 1960 data showed marked improvement for Mexican Americans who, by then, move to an intermediate position between Anglos and blacks.

Not until 1978 did more recent mortality statistics for Mexican Americans become available in published form. Bradshaw and Fonner (1978) computed age-adjusted mortality rates for 1969-1971 for Texas (Table 5.1). They found that overall rates for Spanish-surname men were similar to rates for other white men. Spanish-surname women, however, had death rates that were 19 percent above those for other white females. At age 65 and over, death rates for Spanish-surname males were slightly lower than those for other white males, while rates for Spanish-surname females were clearly higher than those for other white females. Rates for Spanish-surname whites and other whites

Table 5.1 Age-Adjusted Mortality Rates per 100,000 Population for Selected Age Groups by Sex and Ethnicity: Texas, 1969-1971

Age	Spanish-Surname Whites		Non-Spanish-Surname Whites		Nonwhite	
	Males	Females	Males	Females	Males	Females
All Ages	1,256	863	1,273	928	1,477	989
30-44	331	180	283	160	704	383
45-64	1,282	814	1,415	630	2,079	1,375
65 & over	6,941	5,154	7,338	4,516	6,579	4,708

SOURCE: Adapted from Bradshaw and Fonner, 1978.

NOTE: Statistics are directly standardized on Texas non-Spanish-surname white female age distribution.

were considerably lower than rates for nonwhites, except in the case of black men at age 65 and over.

Patterns similar to the ones described above are noted when we examine life expectancy figures for Texas for 1970. Table 5.2 shows that the life expectancy at birth of Spanish-surname men was 67.2 years, compared to 68.1 for other white men. A larger gap existed among females: Spanish-surname females had a life expectancy at birth of 73.4 years, compared to 76.5 for other white women. Blacks were disadvantaged in both sexes with life expectancies of 61.7 and 69.5 years, respectively. At age 65, Spanish-surname men had a life expectancy slightly greater than that of other white men (15.3 vs. 13.5 years) while the life expectancy of Spanish-surname women was slightly lower that that of other white women (16.4 vs. 17.9 years).

Data from California for 1969-1971 show a smaller gap in life expectancy between Spanish-surname persons and other whites. Spanish-surname men had a life expectancy at birth of 68.3 years, compared with 68.7 years for other white men and only 63.5 years for nonwhite men. Similarly, Spanish-surname women had a life expectancy of 75.2 years, compared to 76.0 for other white women and 75.1 for nonwhite women. At ages 40 to 65, male Spanish-surname life expectancy exceeded slightly the male other white life expectancy. The figures for females at these ages were virtually identical in the two ethnic groups. Nonwhites were, again, disadvantaged relative to the other groups, except at age 65.

Table 5.2 Life Expectancy at Selected Ages by Sex and Ethnicity: Texas and California, 1969-1971

State/Age	Spanish-Surname Whites		Non-Spanish-Surname Whites		Nonwhite[a]	
	Males	Females	Males	Females	Males	Females
Texas						
0	67.2	73.4	68.1	76.5	61.7	69.5
20	50.4	56.0	50.5	58.3	45.2	52.3
65	15.3	16.4	13.5	17.9	13.3	16.5
California						
0	68.3	75.2	68.7	76.0	63.5	71.5
15	55.4	62.1	55.5	62.4	51.3	58.9
40	33.4	38.3	32.5	38.6	30.5	36.3
65	14.1	17.4	13.6	17.7	14.5	17.7

SOURCE: Adapted from Siegel and Passel, 1979 (Texas), and Schoen and Nelson, 1981 (California).
[a]Blacks only for California

Data for 1980 show that Mexican Americans may have narrowed the mortality gap even further. Sullivan and her colleagues (1984) have produced estimates of the life expectancy of Mexican Americans in Texas for 1980 (Table 5.3). They present estimates of life expectancy at various ages using four definitions of Mexican Americans. The first column presents estimates for the Spanish-surname population excluding blacks. The second column refers to the Spanish-surname population including all races. These two definitions produce roughly equivalent estimates of life expectancy. Among females, these figures are somewhat lower than those for Anglos (non-Spanish surname persons, excluding blacks) at every age. Among males, however, the figures are lower than those for Anglos only at ages 0 and 20 and are higher at ages 40, 60, and 80. A modified Spanish-surname definition that includes nonblack persons not reporting their surnames produces higher life expectancy figures than for Anglos at every age. Higher life expectancies are also produced by the Spanish-origin definition (fourth column). However, as Sullivan et al. (1984) point out, the Spanish-origin definition is likely to underestimate mortality rates and, consequently, artificially inflate life expectancy figures.

Table 5.3 Life Expectancy at Selected Ages for Hispanics using Alternative Definitions, and Anglos and Blacks: Texas, 1980.

Age	Spanish Surname	Spanish Surname All Races	Spanish Surname+	Spanish Origin	Anglo	Black
			Males			
0	69.6	69.6	72.5	71.0	70.2	64.4
20	51.6	51.7	54.5	52.9	51.9	46.8
40	34.4	34.4	37.0	35.4	33.7	29.8
60	18.3	18.3	20.7	19.1	17.4	16.3
80	7.1	7.1	9.0	7.9	6.8	7.8
			Females			
0	77.1	77.2	81.4	78.8	78.1	73.6
20	52.9	58.6	62.7	60.0	59.4	55.6
40	35.4	39.3	43.4	40.7	40.2	37.1
60	19.1	21.4	25.5	22.7	22.7	21.2
80	7.9	8.0	11.8	9.1	8.7	10.6

SOURCE: Adapted from Sullivan et al. (1984).

NOTE: Denominators derived from U.S. Census as follows:
Spanish Surname: Spanish Surnamed Population, Excluding Blacks
Spanish Surname, All Races: Spanish Surnamed Population, Including All Races
Spanish Surname+: Spanish Surnamed Population Which Reported No Surname, Excluding Blacks
Spanish Origin: Persons Reporting Hispanic Origins, Including All Races
Anglo: Non-Spanish Surnamed Population, Excluding Blacks
Black: Persons Reporting Themselves as Black

It should be clear that the precise estimate of Mexican American mortality is a matter of definition. Yet regardless of the definition employed, the Mexican American mortality situation in Texas in 1980 is much closer to that of Anglos than that of blacks, much like the situation in 1970. Gillespie and Sullivan (1983) calculated age-specific death rates using Spanish-surname numerators and Spanish-surname denominators that show that Spanish-surname males generally have slightly higher mortality than other-surname males until age 54 (Table 5.4). At age 55 and later, their death rates are somewhat lower than those of others. Spanish-surname women, on the other hand, have

Table 5.4 Ratios of Spanish Surname Age-Specific Mortality Rates to Other-Surname Rates by Age and Sex: Texas, 1980

Age Group	Males	Females
Under 5	1.11	1.10
5-9	0.78	1.07
10-14	0.74	1.48
15-19	1.25	0.68
20-24	1.59	0.82
25-29	1.43	0.96
30-34	1.36	0.94
35-39	1.16	0.69
40-44	1.08	0.86
45-49	1.04	0.71
50-54	1.03	0.95
55-59	0.93	0.87
60-64	0.86	1.08
65-69	0.88	1.07
70-74	0.95	1.19
75 and over	0.92	1.04

SOURCE: Adapted from Gillespie and Sullivan, (1983).

lower death rates than other women from age 15 to 59. At age 60 and over, their rates become slightly higher than those of other women. When the overall mortality rates by sex were age-standardized relative to the age structure of "other" Texas males and females, Spanish-surname females had a total death rate of 7.5 per 1,000 compared with 7.0 per 1,000 for other females. Spanish-surname males, however, had a rate of 9.0, which is just below the 9.2 rate for other males.

Table 5.5 presents life expectancy figures for California's Spanish-surname population for 1979-81 with comparable figures for the white and black populations. These figures are slightly higher for the Spanish-surname population than for the white population at every age and for both sexes. As in Texas, blacks have lower figures except at age 85 when a crossover is apparent.

Again, even though there are problems with the Spanish-surname definition, the data from California do not indicate that the Hispanic population there is disadvantaged relative to the white population. Other recent analyses presenting evidence of an overall favorable mortality situation for Hispanics were conducted by Frerichs, Chapman, and Maes (1984) for Los Angeles County and by Shai and Rosenwaike (1987) for metropolitan Chicago.

Table 5.5 Life Expectancy at Selected Ages for Persons of Spanish Surname, Whites, and Blacks: California, 1979-81.

Age	Spanish Surname	Whites	Blacks
	Males		
0	72.0	71.3	65.6
20	53.7	53.0	47.9
40	35.9	34.7	31.1
60	19.3	18.1	16.9
65	15.8	14.7	14.1
70	12.7	11.8	11.6
75	10.1	9.2	9.5
80	7.9	7.1	7.7
85	6.5	5.4	6.6
	Females		
0	79.4	78.4	74.3
20	60.6	59.6	56.2
40	41.4	40.4	37.7
60	23.5	22.8	21.6
65	19.6	18.9	18.3
70	15.9	15.3	15.2
75	12.7	12.1	12.4
80	10.0	9.2	9.9
85	8.1	6.9	8.4

SOURCE: California Center for Health Statistics (1983).

MORTALITY BY CAUSE OF DEATH

Cardiovascular Disease

The limited literature on Hispanic mortality by cause suggests that Southwestern Hispanics have a lower prevalence of cardiovascular diseases than do Anglos or blacks. The literature also suggests that the Hispanic advantage exists only for males. In his San Antonio study, for example, Ellis (1962) found significantly lower mortality from heart diseases among Spanish-surname men than among other white men in 1950. Spanish-surname women, on the other hand, had slightly higher rates than other white women. Similarly, Bradshaw and Fonner (1978) computed a lower age-adjusted death rate from ischemic heart disease

Table 5.6 Age-Adjusted Mortality Rates from Ischemic Heart Disease and Cerebrovascular Disease per 100,000 Population for Selected Age Groups by Sex and Ethnicity: Texas, 1969-1971

Disease/Age	Spanish-Surname Whites		Non-Spanish-Surname Whites		Nonwhite[a]	
	Males	*Females*	*Males*	*Females*	*Males*	*Females*
Ischemic heart disease						
All ages	346.1	225.0	441.4	217.2	382.7	271.8
30-44	30.4	6.7	55.8	9.8	87.4	45.1
45-64	274.1	159.2	530.2	125.7	580.0	363.5
65 and over	2,283.1	1,663.1	2,789.6	1,652.7	2,129.2	1,627.9
Cerebrovascular disease						
All ages	123.9	99.9	130.4	107.7	165.6	159.4
30-44	10.6	10.3	8.1	7.5	33.4	35.1
45-64	95.4	62.5	65.3	46.0	195.2	194.0
65 and over	884.9	787.8	1,003.2	842.1	1,024.2	971.0

SOURCE: Adapted from Bradshaw and Fonner, (1978).

for Spanish-surname men in 1969-1971 in Texas than for other white men (Table 5.6). The rate for Spanish-surname women, however, was higher than the rate for other white women, although the difference was very small (225.0 and 217.2 per 100,000).

Data for California for 1969-1971, presented by Schoen and Nelson (1981), show an overall male Spanish-surname advantage relative to other whites in total cardiovascular mortality. As in Texas, a female Spanish-surname advantage is not observed. Unfortunately, these data are not given separately for heart disease and cerebrovascular diseases. Age-adjusted death rates from cerebrovascular diseases in Texas for 1969-1971 were slightly lower for both male and female Spanish-surname persons and considerably lower than for nonwhites. Kautz (1982) suggested that, although the white/nonwhite differentials in total cardiovascular mortality are due to differences in cerebrovascular mortality, the Spanish-surname/other white differences can be attributed to differences in ischemic heart disease mortality, and this is totally due to differences among males.

Data from New Mexico also show that Hispanics may be advantaged in mortality from diseases of the heart. Buechley, Key, Morris, Morton, and Morgan (1979) found that Spanish-surname males had considerably lower age-adjusted death rates from ischemic heart disease than other white men during 1969-1975. Unfortunately, data for females were not given.

Although cardiovascular diseases are generally diseases of middle and old age, researchers rarely present their findings for different age groups. Bradshaw and Fonner (1978), however, have provided age-adjusted death rates from ischemic heart disease and cerebrovascular disease for broad age groups for 1969-1971 for Texas (Table 5.6). The data show that the advantage of Spanish-surname males relative to other white males in ischemic heart disease mortality is present in each age group. Among people age 65 and over, Spanish-surname males had a death rate of 2,283 per 100,000 compared to a rate of 2,789 for other white men. Non-white men, on the other hand, who have the highest ischemic heart disease rate in younger age groups, have the lowest rate among men at age 65 and over. This is consistent with the low overall death rate of older nonwhites, which may reflect the well-known racial mortality "crossover" phenomenon at advanced ages (see Manton, Poss, & Wing, 1979; Markides, 1983). Among females, there is essentially no difference in ischemic heart disease mortality for the various age groups between Spanish-surname persons and other whites. Nonwhite women, like nonwhite men, have higher death rates than the other two ethnic groups at younger ages but have slightly lower rates at age 65 and over, which suggests the existence of a racial mortality crossover among women.

With regard to cerebrovascular diseases where the overall male Spanish-surname mortality rate is slightly lower than the rate for other whites, Spanish-surname men are disadvantaged at younger ages relative to other whites. However, a crossover is observed in old age, where the Spanish-surname rate is lower than the other white rate (Table 5.6). Nonwhite men are greatly disadvantaged at younger ages relative to Spanish-surname and other white men. At age 65 and over, however, their rate is only slightly higher than the rate for other whites. Spanish-surname females also have higher death rates from cerebrovascular diseases at younger ages but lower rates at age 65 and over. Black women have much higher rates than the other ethnic groups at younger ages. At age 65 and over, their rate is slightly below that for other white women but higher than that for Spanish-surname women.

Data by age were recently presented by Friis, Nanjudappa, Pendergast, and Welsh (1981) from their study in Orange County, California. They found that in 1978 mortality rates from diseases of the heart were considerably lower among Hispanics of both sexes than among non-Hispanics in all age groups. However, since Hispanic rates were computed using Spanish-surname data from death certificates (numerator) and Spanish-origin data for population estimates (denominator), the rate might underestimate the Hispanic mortality from diseases of the heart, particularly at the oldest ages (Gillespie & Sullivan, 1983).

Researchers have recently examined declines in cardiovascular mortality during the 1970's to investigate whether Hispanics have shared in the declines. Kautz, Bradshaw, and Fonner (1981) found that ischemic heart disease and acute myocardial infarction mortality rates showed smaller declines among Spanish-surname persons in Texas from 1970 to 1975 than among other whites and blacks of both sexes. On the other hand, chronic ischemic heart disease mortality increased in importance for all sex-ethnic groups except for Spanish-surname women. In addition, no significant declines in cerebrovascular disease mortality were observed for any of the groups. Stern and Gaskill (1978) observed somewhat similar trends for Bexar County (San Antonio), Texas from 1970 to 1976: Ischemic heart disease mortality rates declined among Spanish-surname males and females and other white males. Acute myocardial infarction death rates declined in all sex-ethnic groups while chronic ischemic heart disease mortality declined only among Spanish-surname women. Finally, no significant declines were observed in cerebrovascular mortality in any of the sex-ethnic groups.

Kautz (1982) observed that the greater declines in overall cardiovascular mortality among blacks, and the relatively smaller declines among Hispanics than among the other two ethnic groups, are bringing the three ethnic groups closer to each other. However, Hispanic rates remain the lowest. Unfortunately, these data are limited to Texas and do not differentiate between the mortality rates of middle-aged and older people.

Stern and his colleagues (1987) have recently presented further evidence on declines in ischemic heart disease mortality for the Spanish-surname population of Texas from 1970 to 1980. These data, which are given by age, were compared with data for non-Hispanic whites. Table 5.7 shows that total ischemic heart disease mortality rates were lower among Hispanic men than among non-Hispanic men at all ages in both 1970 and 1980. However, the overall age-adjusted

Table 5.7 Age-Specific and Age-Adjusted Rates per 100,000 from Chronic Ischemic Heart Disease, Acute Myocardial Infarction, and Ischemic Heart Disease: Texas, 1970 and 1980

Age	Spanish-Surnamed Whites						Other Whites					
	Chronic Ischemic Heart Disease		Acute Myocardial Infarction		Total Ischemic Heart Disease		Chronic Ischemic Heart Disease		Acute Myocardial Infarction		Total Ischemic Heart Disease	
	1970	1980	1970	1980	1970	1980	1970	1980	1970	1980	1970	1980
Males												
35-44	7.3	11.8	36.5	25.2	43.8	37.0	19.8	18.1	59.9	31.7	79.7	49.8
45-54	40.9	53.6	152.6	115.9	193.5	169.5	81.3	74.5	236.2	136.9	317.5	211.4
55-64	155.6	156.9	435.5	299.2	591.1	456.1	224.5	191.4	588.5	363.1	813.0	554.5
65-74	459.4	450.3	917.5	762.6	1376.9	1212.9	574.4	488.7	1194.0	810.6	1768.4	1299.3
75+	1716.6	1542.5	1888.0	1439.7	3604.6	2982.2	1987.7	1772.9	2315.6	1776.3	4303.3	3549.2
Age-Adjusted	268.1	256.1	450.5	344.7	718.6	600.8	338.7	297.3	592.1	403.4	930.8	700.7
Females												
35-44	3.3	2.5	7.0	3.2	10.3	5.7	4.7	4.4	9.5	5.8	14.2	10.2
45-54	22.5	13.3	38.8	26.5	61.3	39.8	17.7	16.0	39.9	28.9	57.6	44.9
55-64	103.2	65.5	171.5	120.7	274.7	186.2	66.4	58.9	145.4	102.8	211.8	161.7
65-74	358.0	251.7	557.9	353.4	915.9	605.1	265.3	216.6	450.1	320.5	715.4	537.1
75+	1536.6	1324.3	1289.6	6921.8	2826.2	2246.1	1657.3	1361.9	1468.0	1081.2	3125.3	2443.1
Age-Adjusted	219.5	173.9	247.2	168.8	466.7	342.7	207.6	171.9	242.6	175.7	450.2	347.6

SOURCE: Adapted from Stern (1987).

difference between the groups was lower in 1980 owing to steeper declines among non-Hispanic men. Overall age-adjusted rates were comparable in Hispanic and non-Hispanic women in both years. Again, steep declines were observed for both ethnic groups in total ischemic heart disease mortality from 1970 to 1980.

Table 5.7 shows that the picture for acute myocardial infarction mortality is quite similar to that for total ischemic heart disease mortality: the overall Hispanic male advantage was reduced from 1970 to 1980 by steeper declines in non-Hispanic male rates, while no significant ethnic differences were observed among women in either 1970 or 1980. Again, the rates were much lower in 1980 than in 1970. Finally, Table 5.7 shows that Hispanic men were advantaged in chronic ischemic heart disease mortality at every age in both 1970 and 1980. However, this advantage narrowed considerably during the decade owing to negligible declines in the rates for Hispanic men in the face of relatively marked declines among non-Hispanic white men. Women in both ethnic groups exhibited significant declines during the decade, but no significant ethnic differences are observed in chronic ischemic heart disease mortality among women in either year. These data, in sum, suggest that Hispanic men continue to be advantaged in ischemic heart disease mortality but at a lower rate. Hispanic women, on the other hand do not exhibit an advantage over other white women.

Frerichs and his colleagues (1984) have shown that Hispanics had lower overall adjusted mortality rates from major cardiovascular diseases than whites in Los Angeles County in 1980. Unfortunately, these rates were not presented separately by sex to examine whether this advantage is observed only among men as is the case in Texas (note that 1978 Orange County data discussed earlier showed both a male and a female Hispanic advantage in coronary heart disease mortality). Frerichs et al. also computed lower mortality rates from cerebrovascular diseases among Hispanics than among whites. Again, no sex (or age) comparisons were presented. Similar findings were found by Shai and Rosenwaike (1987) in the Chicago area.

The apparent advantage of Hispanics in cardiovascular mortality begs for an explanation. National data show that Hispanics (Mexican Americans) may have the lowest systolic and diastolic blood pressures while blacks have the highest (Table 5.8). The Hispanic advantage also exists among persons 65-74, but it is slight. Moreover, it is not consistent for all age groups. The study by Friis et al. (1981) in Orange County found no differences between Hispanics and non-Hispanics in systolic and diastolic blood pressure. Christensen, Stallones Insell,

Table 5.8 Systolic and Diastolic Blood Pressures (mmHg) in Persons 18 to 74 Years of Age by Ethnicity and Age: United States, 1971-1974

Pressure/Age	White	Spanish/ Mexican American	Black
Systolic			
18-24	119.3 ± 13.6	114.8 ± 13.0	117.5 ± 15.2
25-34	120.4 ± 14.5	119.4 ± 14.0	125.2 ± 15.9
35-44	124.8 ± 17.0	123.3 ± 17.4	132.8 ± 20.7
45-54	132.8 ± 21.1	134.5 ± 17.2	146.4 ± 32.3
55-64	141.3 ± 23.1	142.4 ± 24.5	149.7 ± 26.1
65-74	149.2 ± 24.6	147.9 ± 20.4	159.3 ± 28.6
Diastolic			
18-24	73.8 ± 10.4	70.6 ± 8.9	74.2 ± 11.0
25-34	77.5 ± 10.6	76.7 ± 9.6	81.0 ± 12.9
35-44	81.7 ± 11.9	79.7 ± 11.2	88.5 ± 13.3
45-54	84.9 ± 13.1	85.0 ± 10.1	92.7 ± 16.2
55-64	86.3 ± 12.2	86.3 ± 8.7	91.7 ± 14.0
65-74	85.5 ± 12.7	82.0 ± 10.7	90.6 ± 15.1

SOURCE: National Center for Health Statistics, 1977.
NOTE: Figures are means ± standard deviations.

Gotto, and Taunton (1981) found no differences in either systolic or diastolic blood pressure levels between Mexican American and other white men in Houston. Mexican American women, however, had higher levels than other white women but lower levels than black women. These findings held in all adult age groups. Data from Starr County, Texas (Hanis, Ferrell, & Schull, 1985) showed that rates of definite hypertension were lower among Mexican Americans from that county than for the U.S. white population in all age groups (from 18 to 74) and for both sexes. However, rates for borderline hypertension were uniformly higher among Mexican Americans yielding no ethnic differences in the overall prevalence of hypertension. Data from the San Antonio Heart Study (Franco, et al., 1985) suggested that in general, Mexican Americans tended to have lower rates of hypertension than Anglos, but these differences were not statistically significant. However, hypertension rates decreased from lower to higher socioeconomic status neighborhoods in both ethnic groups. Finally, data from Laredo showed no significant differences in mean systolic and diastolic pressure between Mexican American men participating in the study and U.S. whites. Mexican American women, however, were found to have slightly lower systolic and diastolic blood pressures than U.S. white women in most age groups. In sum, there is no consistent evidence that blood pressure levels of Mexican Americans of both sexes and all age groups are significantly different from those of other whites. Thus, any advantage Mexican Americans may enjoy in cardiovascular disease mortality cannot be explained by lower blood pressure levels or lower rates of hypertension.

A California study found that Mexican Americans had lower serum cholesterol than whites, but the difference was slight (National Center for Health Statistics, 1978). Friis et al. (1981), on the other hand, found higher serum cholesterol among Hispanic men than among non-Hispanic men and slightly lower cholesterol among Hispanic women than among non-Hispanic women. Christensen et al. (1981) found higher overall cholesterol among Mexican American men than other white men in Houston. Mexican American women, on the other hand, had lower total cholesterol than other white women.

National data show that Hispanics smoke and drink less than other whites (National Center for Health Statistics, 1980a), findings that are confirmed by the Orange County study (Friis et al., 1981). With regard to smoking, the situation may be changing. A recent literature review (Marcus & Crane, 1985) and a San Antonio study (Markides, Coreil, & Ray, 1987) show that smoking rates among Mexican American men are equal to, if not greater than, those of other men, although Mexican Americans appear to smoke fewer cigarettes. Mexican American women continue to smoke at lower rates than other women. The evidence on alcohol consumption suggests that Mexican American men might be less frequent drinkers than other men, but they tend to contain a disproportionate number of excessive drinkers. Mexican American women are lighter drinkers than women in the general population, but have been found to drink more with greater acculturation into the larger society (Caetano, 1983; Gilbert & Cervantes, 1986; Markides, Krause, & Mendes de Leon, 1988). Finally, Hispanics are more obese and less physically active than other whites (National Center for Health Statistics, 1980a) and are generally less likely to engage in life-styles that promote cardiovascular health (Castro, Baezconde-Garbanati, & Beltran, 1985; Hazuda, Stern, Gaskill, Haffner, & Gardner, 1983). As we will also see below, Mexican Americans have considerably higher rates of diabetes than other whites, another known risk factor for cardiovascular disease. Obviously, no clear factors emerge from the available evidence that might explain the apparent Mexican American advantage in cardiovascular mortality.

Cancer

Hispanics also appear to be advantaged in major cancers (Tables 5.9 and 5.10). The relative advantage for Hispanics is most pronounced for cancers of the lung, breast, colon-rectum, prostate, and pancreas. Higher mortality rates among Hispanics, on the other hand, are found for malignancies of the cervix, stomach, liver, and gall bladder. Cancer incidence data for Texas (McDonald & Heinze, 1978) and New Mexico (Young, 1982) confirm these ethnic mortality patterns. Examination of cancer rates by sex and site points to possible etiological mechanisms.

Data for 1969-1971 for Texas show that, in contrast to males, Hispanic females have a total cancer mortality rate that is slightly higher than that of white females but lower than that of black females. This excess female cancer mortality is present in the 45-64 age group as well as in the 65 and older group (Table 5.9). Spanish-surname men, on the other hand, have a lower cancer death rate at every age, including 65 years and over. Blacks are clearly disadvantaged at younger ages, but in old age their cancer death rates are just below the rates of other whites.

If we look at site-specific death rates, some interesting patterns emerge. For cancers of the trachea and lung, Hispanic females fare slightly worse than the comparison groups, yet most of the excess deaths occur at older ages (Table 5.9). Hispanic males of all ages die of lung cancer at much lower rates than other white males (see also Buechley, Dunn, Linden, & Breslow, 1957; Lee, Roberts, & Labarthe, 1976; Menck et al., 1975). The relative disadvantage of black men at younger ages becomes an advantage at age 65 and over.

Rosenwaike (1988) has recently presented data on cancer mortality for the Mexican-born population of the United States for 1979-1981. These data show an advantage of the Mexican-born population relative to all whites in most cancers except in the cases of stomach and liver cancers, and cancer of the cervix where Mexican-born females had rates twice those of white females (see also Peters, Thomas, Hagan, Mack, & Henderson, 1986). In addition, Mexican-born females had a slightly higher mortality rate from cancer of the pancreas. Similar findings were obtained in a recent study of the Mexican-born population of Illinois (Mullin & Anderson, 1988). These findings overall

Table 5.9 Age-Adjusted Cancer Mortality Rates per 100,000 Population for Selected Age Groups by Sex and Ethnicity: Texas, 1969-1971

Type of Cancer/Age	Spanish-Surname Whites		Non-Spanish-Surname Whites		Nonwhite	
	Males	*Females*	*Males*	*Females*	*Males*	*Females*
All neoplasms						
All ages	185.6	147.7	218.0	133.0	238.9	152.4
30-44	32.4	48.3	42.3	49.1	59.6	68.2
45-64	216.6	235.4	320.0	223.9	440.5	308.2
65 and over	1,136.7	748.5	1,211.4	640.7	1,151.5	621.4
Trachea and lung						
All ages	43.9	14.1	70.2	13.0	63.4	11.3
30-44	4.9	2.2	11.6	5.8	18.4	4.9
45-64	53.1	20.4	134.3	29.6	151.3	24.8
65 and over	277.9	82.3	346.6	49.5	243.1	
Breast						
All ages	—	19.5	—	24.5	—	24.5
30-44	—	13.2	—	14.3	—	24.5
45-64	—	42.0	—	55.9	—	57.5
65 and over	—	72.3	—	87.3	—	78.0
Cervix/uteri						
All ages	—	12.6	—	5.4	—	15.2
30-44	—	8.0	—	5.0	—	12.1
45-64	—	28.1	—	9.8	—	37.5
65 and over	—	42.3	—	20.3	—	42.4

SOURCE: Adapted from Bradshaw and Fonner, (1978).

NOTE: Statistics are directly standardized on the Texas non-Spanish-surname white female age distribution.

suggest that the cancer mortality rates of the Mexican-born population, particularly males, may be slightly more favorable than those of the Mexican American population.

The data on the Mexican-born population of the United States are also showing an advantage among females in lung cancer, which is inconsistent with earlier data from Texas. However, data from Los Angeles and New Mexico do show an advantage in overall lung cancer mortality for Hispanic women relative to Anglo women making the picture inconclusive (Newell & Mills, 1987). Newell and Mills have

Table 5.10 Colo-Rectal, Pancreatic, and Prostatic Cancer Mortality Rates per 100,000 Population Selected Age Groups by Sex and Ethnicity: Texas, 1980

Type of Cancer/Age	Spanish-Surname Whites		Non-Spanish-Surname Whites		Nonwhite	
	Males	*Females*	*Males*	*Females*	*Males*	*Females*
Colo-rectal						
35-54	5	3	10	7	9	8
55-74	34	24	68	54	69	63
75 and over	98	85	244	215	195	295
Pancreatic						
35-54	5	4	5	3	14	2
55-74	28	30	37	23	57	40
75 and over	93	50	101	85	112	61
Prostatic						
35-54	1.2	—	0.6	—	1.3	—
55-74	39	—	52	—	87	—
75 and over	224	—	364	—	516	—

SOURCE: Bureau of Vital Statistics, Texas Department of Health, (1981).

suggested that the earlier higher lung cancer rates of older Hispanic women may have been the result of high smoking rates at an earlier age during the time of the Mexican Revolution. This is supported by a recent study in New Mexico that found that lung cancer mortality among older Hispanic women has declined in recent years (Samet, Key, Kutvirt, & Wiggins, 1988).

Data from Denver show that lung cancer rates for the Denver area were lower in both sexes among Spanish-surname persons than among other whites in 1969-1971. However, the female gap was rather small (Savitz, 1986). These rates increased significantly in all sex-ethnic groups by 1979-1981 with the relative advantage of Hispanic males diminishing considerably. This convergence was also observed in other cancer rates, leading Savitz to conclude that this convergence is the result of higher smoking rates among Hispanics as well as the adoption of the more general life-styles of the larger society.

As we have seen previously, there is evidence that smoking rates among Hispanic men are equal to or even greater than the rates for other men (Marcus & Crane, 1985; Markides et al., 1987). Since traditionally lower smoking rates among Hispanics have been used to partially explain the advantage of Hispanics in lung cancer, the recent increase in smoking can be expected to narrow or eliminate this advantage in the near future.

Mortality differences by ethnicity for breast and cervical cancer suggest a potential association with reproductive behavior (Menck et al., 1975). Mexican American females have earlier and higher fertility than do women in other ethnic groups, a factor that may partly explain the lower risk for breast cancer and the elevated risk for cervical cancer found in this group (Table 5.8). Early onset of sexual relations is associated with cervical cancer (Rotkin, 1973; Terris, Wilson, Smith, Strung, & Nelson, 1967), and breast cancer has been linked to early childbearing and high fertility (MacMahon et al., 1970; Research Group for Population-Based Cancer Registration, 1976). (See also Newell & Mills, 1987.)

A possible nutritional link is also suggested in the combination of lower risk for breast and colon cancer among Hispanics (Tables 5.9 and 5.10). This trend appears to be consistent for both sexes across all age groups. Newell and Boutwell (1981) hypothesized that dietary patterns, perhaps involving levels of fat and fiber consumption, may explain the relative advantage for breast and colon cancer mortality among Mexican Americans. (See also Newell & Mills, 1987.)

Finally, a possible genetic influence in ethnic cancer rates is suggested by the fact that populations with partial Indian ancestry, including Mexican Americans, have rates for most cancers that are intermediate between those for Anglos and tribes with generally full Indian heritage (Sievers & Fisher, 1983). Data from New Mexico support the case for a proportionate genetic contribution to cancer mortality, with the strongest argument made in studies of gall bladder cancer among that state's tri-ethnic population (Devor & Buechley, 1980; Morris, Buechley, Key, & Morgan, 1978).

Diabetes

Noninsulin-dependent diabetes mellitus (NIDDM) is a major health problem in middle-aged and older people. Prevalence rates for non-insulin-dependent diabetes are two to five times greater among Mexican Americans than among the general U.S. population (Hanis et al., 1983; Stern, Gaskill, Hazuda, Gardner, & Haffner, 1983). Data for 1969-1971 for Texas show that mortality from diabetes was much higher among Spanish-surname persons than among other whites or blacks in both sexes and at every age. Elevated risk for diabetes is found among males and females at all ages; however, the largest is among older Hispanic women (Bradshaw & Fonner, 1978). Data for 1980 from California also show much higher mortality rates among Spanish- surname persons at every age after 45 (California Center for Health Statistics, 1983). The same was observed among Mexican immigrants in the Chicago area (Shai & Rosenwaike, 1987).

Obesity has been studied as a possible risk factor underlying these differences. High rates of diabetes and obesity are characteristic of economically disadvantaged groups in general, and Stern et al. (1981) found elevated rates of both diabetes and obesity among Mexican Americans in Laredo, Texas. More recent findings from the San Antonio Heart Study (Stern et al., 1983), however, show that obesity alone cannot account for the high rate of diabetes. After controlling for social class and obesity, the risk of diabetes among Mexican Americans of both sexes was even greater than without such controls. It is further hypothesized that obesity and certain patterns of body fat may be associated with diabetes (Haffner, 1987). Mexican Americans are characterized by a high prevalence of generalized adiposity and a more unfavorable body-fat distribution (Haffner, Stern, Hazuda, Pugh, & Patterson, 1987). Studies by Haffner and his associates (1986, 1987) have indicated that both central and upper body adiposity are associated with higher rates of NIDDM in Mexican Americans. However, even after adjusting for greater overall and more centralized adiposity, the greater prevalence of NIDDM in Mexican Americans remains.

As with cancer, it appears that genetic factors at least partially explain the prevalence of diabetes among Hispanics. High rates of diabetes are found among American Indians, and those tribes with close to 100 percent native genes, such as the Pima, have the highest rates of all. Moreover, a correspondence between genetic admixture and diabetes has been reported in studies comparing tribes of varying genetic makeup (Brousseau, Eelkema, Crawford, & Abe, 1979). Given the variable presence of Native American genes in the Hispanic population, one would expect genetic factors to influence diabetes in proportion to hereditary affinity. Research conducted in San Antonio has also uncovered that a degree of Native American admixture is related to diabetes prevalence among Mexican Americans even after other factors are taken into consideration (Gardner et al., 1984; Relethford, Stern, Gaskill, & Hazuda, 1983; Stern et al., 1983).

As with other populations, such as the Pima Indians, who are at high risk for NIDDM, Mexican Americans have more hyperinsulinemia than can be accounted for by their obesity and pattern of fat distribution. One possible explanation for the hyperinsulinemia is prolonged insulin secretion, secondary to increased insulin resistance, which could lead to islet cell decomposition and eventually to diabetes (Haffner, 1987).

Given the high rates of NIDDM in Mexican Americans, complications of the disease are an important and under-investigated health issue. In a study by Pugh and her associates (1988), the age-specific incidence of diabetes-related end-stage renal disease as well as renal disease from other etiologies were computed using the 1980 census for the state of Texas and a data base from the Texas Kidney Health Program. For diabetes-related end-stage renal disease, Mexican Americans have an incidence ratio of six compared to non-Hispanic whites. This excess is higher than would be expected on the basis of their underlying prevalence of NIDDM. Similarly, the incidence of hypertension-related end-stage renal disease in Mexican Americans is 2.5 times greater than in non-Hispanic whites, which is also unexpected given the lower prevalence of hypertension in this population. In addition, Mexican Americans have rates of glomerulonephritic end-stage renal disease and end-stage renal disease of unknown etiology in excess of what might be predicted from rates of existing diseases.

When looking at age-specific incidences, Mexican Americans and non-Hispanic whites until the age of 40 have similar risks for developing the diabetes-related end-stage renal disease. After the age of 40, the risk rises faster for Mexican Americans while the age-specific curve for non-Hispanic whites is almost flat. There are also excessive rates of hypertension-related end-stage renal disease in all older age groups.

Pugh, Stern, Haffner, Eifler, and Zapata (1988) recognized this is an initial investigation in this population and the potential for some disease misclassification. However, the rates are similar to those found in a study by Eggers, Connerton, & McMullon (1984). The explanation for these excesses may be partially found in a higher prevalence of risk factors in the Mexican American population for the development of end-stage renal disease including level of glycemic control, duration of the diabetes, coexistent hypertension, and proteinuria.

Other Diseases

In addition to diabetes, Hispanics appear to be disadvantaged in other diseases. Data from Texas for 1969-1971 showed that Spanish-surname whites were considerably more likely to die from infectious and parasitic diseases, influenza and pneumonia, and accidents and all violent deaths than were other whites. Their death rate from infectious and parasitic diseases was even higher than the rate for nonwhites, as was the female rate from influenza and pneumonia. The male Spanish-surname death rate from influenza and pneumonia was slightly lower than the nonwhite rate, and death rates from accidents and violence were considerably lower among Spanish-surname persons than among nonwhites.

Data from California for 1969-1971 are in general agreement with the data from Texas. Spanish-surname persons had higher age-adjusted death rates than other whites from infectious and parasitic diseases, from influenza and pneumonia, and from accidents and violence. Spanish-surname women, however, had lower death rates than other white women from causes other than motor vehicle accidents and violence (Schoen & Nelson, 1981).

Table 5.11 shows ethnic differences in mortality from the diseases under discussion for broad age groups for Texas in 1969-1971. The Spanish-surname disadvantage in infectious and parasitic diseases relative to other whites is evident at every age, including persons 65 years old and over, where the death rate is approximately three times as great and holds for both sexes. The Spanish-surname disadvantage relative to nonwhites is also significant in old age, where the Spanish-surname death rate is twice as high as the nonwhite rate among men and two and a half times as high among women.

The Spanish-surname to other white disadvantage in mortality from influenza and pneumonia is slight among men, including those age 65 and over. Among women, however, the disadvantage is notable and exists. at each age. The Spanish-surname death rate from influenza/pneumonia is considerably lower than the nonwhite rate at ages 30-64 but is higher at age 65 and over. This is observed in both sexes (Table 5.11).

The Spanish-surname to other white disadvantage in male mortality from accidents and violence is notable at ages 30-44, but is only slight among persons at age 45 and older. A female Spanish-surname ad-

Table 5.11 Adjusted Mortality Rates per 100,000 Population from Infectious and Parasitic Diseases, Influenza and Pneumonia, and Accidents and Violence for Selected Age Groups by Age and Ethnicity: Texas, 1969-1971

Disease/Age	Spanish-Surname Whites		Non-Spanish-Surname Whites		Nonwhite	
	Males	*Females*	*Males*	*Females*	*Males*	*Females*
Infectious and parasitic diseases						
All ages	31.8	18.7	10.2	6.3	22.1	12.7
30-44	7.1	8.0	2.6	1.7	13.0	6.3
45-64	26.0	14.9	11.8	6.5	27.3	16.7
65 and over	150.9	73.1	46.6	25.6	74.0	30.3
Influenza and pneumonia						
All ages	49.3	36.8	41.6	25.6	54.0	30.7
30-44	4.1	7.3	4.1	4.0	20.8	10.4
45-64	27.9	17.4	26.0	13.4	55.6	27.9
65 and over	310.1	224.0	281.5	169.6	246.8	139.3
Accidents and violence						
All ages	123.8	37.6	108.6	47.6	183.6	56.3
30-44	157.5	30.9	111.7	43.0	315.1	66.2
45-64	142.9	32.9	138.8	51.3	245.5	55.8
65 and over	259.6	100.9	243.7	129.9	197.6	98.1

SOURCE: Adapted from Bradshaw and Fonner, (1978).
NOTE: Statistics are directly standardized on Texas non-Spanish-surname white female age distribution.

vantage is noted at every age. At ages 30-64, Spanish-surname mortality from accidents and violence is considerably lower than the rate for nonwhites. At age 65 and over, however, the Spanish-surname rate is higher than the nonwhite rate among males while no difference is noted among women (Table 5.11).

Data from New Mexico for 1976-1978 are available for selected causes of death (State of New Mexico, 1980). They show that mortality from influenza and pneumonia is lower among Spanish-surname men at ages 35-64 than among other whites of similar age. At ages 65-74, the rate is higher among Spanish-surname men but becomes lower again after age 75. Spanish-surname women also have lower death rates from influenza and pneumonia at ages 35-64 and slightly higher death rates at age 65 and over.

New Mexico data also show that Spanish-surname men have higher death rates than other whites from accidents and violence until age 54, and lower rates at age 55 and over. As in Texas and California, however, Spanish-surname women have lower death rates from accidents and violence than other white women. More recent data from the Chicago area confirm high mortality among Mexican immigrants from homicide, pneumonia, and infectious diseases (Shai & Rosenwaike, 1987).

Fracture of the proximal femur (hip) not due to severe trauma is a major medical problem in persons over the age of 50, causing pain, incapacitation, and increased mortality. Due to a hypothesized connection between the loss of estrogen and the development of osteoporosis, postmenopausal women appear to be at particular risk (Kreiger, Kelsey, Holford, & O'Connor, 1982). However, the incidence of hip fractures varies widely among ethnic groups, with little known about the risk of fractures in Hispanics (Bauer, 1988).

In studies in Texas, the incidence of hip fractures among Hispanics, blacks, and non-Hispanic whites living in Bexar County (San Antonio) were calculated for 1980 by Bauer (1988), who confirmed earlier case control findings (Bauer, Diehl, Barton et al., 1986) that Mexican Americans and blacks of both sexes had lower risks of hip fractures than whites. Hip fracture incidence in women in all three ethnic groups increased rapidly in the sixth and seventh decades, coinciding with an anticipated onset of menopause. This supports the hypothesis that onset of menopause is associated with an increase in the risk of hip fractures. However, as Bauer suggested, because of the relatively low risk of fracture in Mexican American women, the benefits of postmenopausal estrogen therapy for these women may not outweigh the expense or risks involved in the treatment (Haber, 1985). Obviously more research is needed in this area, as well as on other common diseases of old age, about which little is known for Hispanics. A recent study of Hispanic elderly in Los Angeles County (Lopez-Aqueres, Kemp, Plopper, Staples, & Brummel-Smith, 1984) has found evidence of high rates of cognitive impairment and organic brain syndrome, for example, but no direct comparisons with non-Hispanics were available.

FUNCTIONAL HEALTH INDICATORS

Most of the information presented thus far is based on relatively objective data obtained from death certificates and clinical assessments. Such data are useful in that they provide "disease" or "medical" models of the health of populations, but they say little about how populations perceive and cope with disease, illness, and disability. "Functional" models define health in terms of a person's ability to function. Such models have been particularly popular in gerontology. Their proponents believe that "the things that an old person can do, or thinks he can do, are useful indicators of both how healthy he is and the services he will require" (Shanas & Maddox, 1976, p. 597).

Shanas and Maddox (1976) suggested that the medical and functional models are not irreconcilable as evidenced by efforts to compare physical examination findings with self-reports by older people. Such efforts have shown moderate associations between physical examination findings or other objective health indicators and self-ratings (e.g., Fillenbaum, 1979; Maddox & Douglass, 1973), suggesting that the two represent different, albeit related, dimensions of health.

Elderly Hispanics have been found to rate their health as poorer than Anglos but better than blacks. National data for 1976-1977, for example, show 24.4 percent of Spanish-origin elderly, compared with 30.9 percent of white and 20.3 percent of black elderly, rating their health as "excellent." Conversely, 11.4 percent of Spanish-origin, 7.4 percent of white, and 16.7 percent of black elderly rated their health as "poor" (National Center for Health Statistics, 1980a, p. 42). Similar findings comparing elderly Mexican Americans and Anglos in San Antonio were obtained by Markides and Martin (1983) (See also the review by Newton, 1980.) The extent to which the lower self-ratings of health by elderly Hispanics relative to elderly Anglos (as well as their better self-ratings relative to elderly blacks) reflect their more "objective" health status can be ascertained by examining data from the 1976 Health Interview Survey (Moy & Wilder, 1978). Table 5.12 shows that Spanish-origin persons reported lower age-adjusted limitation of activity due to chronic conditions and fewer days lost from work per currently employed person than the total and black populations.

On the other hand, persons of Spanish origin reported slightly greater restricted activity and bed disability days than the total, but less than the black population. They also reported slightly fewer doctor visits and short-stay hospital episodes than the total population, al-

Table 5.12 Percentage of Population with Selected Health Characteristics by National Origin or Race and Age: United States, 1976

Characteristics	Total Population	Spanish Origin[a]	Black[a]	Other
Limitation of activity due to chronic conditions				
All ages[b]	14.3	13.5	17.4	14.0
Under 17	3.7	2.8	3.7	3.9
17-44	8.9	7.7	10.5	8.7
45-64	24.3	23.5	32.3	23.4
65 and over	45.4	34.9	52.8	44.6
Doctor visit in past year				
All ages[b]	75.5	70.4	74.2	76.2
Under 17	74.2	67.6	67.6	76.2
17-44	75.4	69.8	76.9	75.6
45-64	75.2	71.2	76.1	75.2
65 and over	80.0	79.4	78.8	80.2
Short-stay hospital episode in past year				
All ages[b]	10.6	10.4	10.6	10.6
Under 17	5.5	5.4	4.7	5.7
17-44	11.4	12.0	13.5	11.0
45-64	12.5	10.8	12.0	12.6
65 and over	18.3	17.1	12.9	18.8
Days of restricted activity per person per year				
All ages[b]	18.2	20.3	23.3	17.6
Under 17	11.0	14.3	7.5	11.3
17-44	14.2	12.9	19.1	13.6
45-64	25.4	26.5	39.1	23.8
65 and over	40.0	53.1	52.5	38.4
Days of bed disability per person per year				
All ages[b]	7.1	9.3	9.9	6.6
Under 17	5.1	7.8	3.9	5.0
17-44	5.6	7.0	8.5	5.1
45-64	8.9	10.5	16.9	8.0
65 and over	15.1	20.5	18.5	14.6

(*continued*)

Table 5.12 (Continued)

Characteristics	Total Population	Spanish Origin[a]	Black[a]	Other
Days lost from work per currently employed person per year				
All ages under 17[b]	5.3	5.0	7.4	5.1
17-44	5.0	4.6	7.7	4.8
45-64	6.1	6.1	7.2	6.0
65 and over	4.0	3.7[c]	4.0[c]	4.0
Days of bed disability per person per year				
All ages[b]	7.1	9.3	9.9	6.6
Under 17	5.1	7.8	3.9	5.0
17-44	5.6	7.0	8.5	5.1
45-64	8.9	10.5	16.9	8.0
65 and over	15.1	20.5	18.5	14.6
Days lost from work per currently employed person per year				
All ages under 17[b]	5.3	5.0	7.4	5.1
17-44	5.0	4.6	7.7	4.8
45-64	6.1	6.1	7.2	6.0
65 and over	4.0	3.7[c]	4.0[c]	4.0

SOURCE: Moy and Wilder (1978).
a. Persons reported as both Spanish origin and black are included in both categories.
b. Figures for all were age-adjusted by the direct method to the age distribution of the civilian noninstitutionalized population or that of the currently employed population.
c. Figure does not meet standards of reliability and validity.

though it is not clear whether the last two variables are indicators of health status or of health care utilization. Among persons at age 65 and over, there is virtually no difference between Spanish-origin persons and the total population on activity limitation due to chronic conditions and doctor visits. Slightly fewer Spanish-origin elderly reported a short-stay hospital episode than all elderly. On the other hand, they reported more days of restricted activity and bed disability than the total population. Finally, Spanish-origin elderly reported fewer days lost from work, although this figure was based on too few cases to yield a reliable estimate.

Additional data are also available from the National Health Interview Survey conducted in 1978-80 (National Center for Health Statistics, 1984). They confirm previous findings that with the exception of dental problems, persons of Mexican origin (who mostly reside in the southwestern states) appear to be advantaged relative to blacks, but are quite similar to other whites on most health indicators. These data, however, reveal interesting patterns by age. Although persons of Mexican origin report fewer disability and restricted activity days under age 45, they report more such days at age 45 and over. These differences are particularly wide at the 65 and older age group. The elderly Mexican origin group also report more activity limitation due to chronic conditions than do other whites in this age group.

The above figures on the functional health indicators of the Hispanic elderly are generally consistent with their lower self-ratings of health relative to elderly Anglos and higher self-ratings relative to elderly blacks. They are not, however, consistent with the lower prevalence of cancer and cardiovascular disease.

CONCLUSION

Little is known about the health status of Hispanics in the Southwest and even less is known about the health status of older Hispanics, a small but rapidly growing component of this population. The data presented here are largely from official records (vital statistics and census enumerations). Problems of linking the two for studying the health and demographic characteristics of Hispanics are well-known (see, e.g., Hernandez, Estrada, & Alvirez, 1973; Trevino, 1982), and while community surveys avoid such issues, they, too, have their problems in identifying Hispanic populations (Hayes-Bautista, 1980).

If anything can be deduced about the health status of Hispanics from the evidence presented here, it is that the health status of Hispanics in the Southwest falls between that of other whites and that of blacks. This appears to be also true for older Hispanics. However, Hispanics appear to have lower death rates from diseases of the heart and cancer, an advantage that appears to be confined to men. Primary prevention factors might be involved, but they do not appear to explain this advantage. Why it occurs only among men remains a mystery at this time.

The nonwhite disadvantage in overall mortality as well as in cardiovascular and cancer mortality disappears or even reverses itself at advanced ages. Although poor quality data on older blacks might be a factor, scholars have speculated that high early mortality among blacks results in a kind of selective survival to advanced ages, particularly after age 75 (see Manton et al., 1979; Markides, 1983. See also the introductory chapter in this book). The absence of this kind of cross-over in the mortality rates of Southwestern Hispanics and other whites may result from the fact that overall Hispanic mortality rates are not markedly lower than those of other whites.

Available data also make it clear that Hispanics at all ages are disadvantated relative to others in diabetes mortality (and also incidence) and in mortality from infectious and parasitic diseases and from influenza/pneumonia, a disadvantage shared with American Indian groups. It appears that genetic factors are partly responsible for the diabetes problem.

Research thus far has not clearly demonstrated how socioeconomic and cultural factors affect the health status of older Hispanics. For example, little is known about how the Hispanic diet affects the incidence of certain diseases. Data on such factors as smoking and alcohol consumption are too sketchy to indicate how they might affect health, although new data are becoming constantly available. There is often discussion about the protective qualities of the Hispanic family, which is thought to shield individuals from stress to a larger extent than families in other groups, but this notion remains unsupported by systematic analysis.

As Hispanic are becoming more acculturated into the larger society, they appear to be adopting some of its values and practices that might affect their health. Alcohol consumption, for example, appears to increase with acculturation among women (Caetano, 1983; Markides et al, 1988). How these changes will affect the health status and health needs of older Hispanics in the years to come is not clear. Fortunately, data from the recently completed Hispanic Health and Nutrition Examination Survey, conducted by the National Center for Health Statistics, are now available on a large sample of Hispanics (including people to age 74), and a number of investigators are currently analyzing them. This study, however, does have a number of limitations, including too few older people, for certain analyses. Large scale epidemiologic investigations in specific communities are necessary for improving our understanding of what happens to the health status of Hispanics as they get older.

REFERENCES

Andersen, R., Lewis, S. Z., Giachello, A. L., Aday, L. A., & Chin, G. (1981). Access to medical care among the Hispanic population of the Southwestern United States. *Journal of Health and Social Behavior, 22*, 78-89.

Bauer, R. L. (1988). Ethnic differences in hip fractures: A reduced incidence in Mexican Americans. *American Journal of Epidemiology, 127*, 145-149.

Bauer, R. L., Diehl, A. K., Barton, S. A., et al. (1986). Risk of postmenopausal hip fractures in Mexican American women. *American Journal of Public Health, 76*, 1020-1021.

Black, W. C., & Key, C. R. (1980). Epidemiologic pathology in New Mexico's tri-ethnic population. *Pathology Annual, 15*, 181-194.

Bradshaw, B. S., & Fonner, E., Jr. (1978). The mortality of Spanish-surnamed persons in Texas: 1969-1971. In F. D. Bean & W. P. Frisbie (Eds.), *The demography of racial and ethnic groups* (pp. 261-282). New York: Academic Press.

Brosseau, J. D., Eelkema, R. C., Crawford, A. C., & Abe, C. A. (1979). Diabetes among the three affiliated tribes: Correlation with degree of Indian inheritance. *American Journal of Public Health, 69*, 1277-1278.

Buechley, R. W., Dunn, J. E., Jr., Linden, G., & Breslow, L. (1957). Excessive lung cancer mortality rates among Mexican-American women in California. *Cancer, 10*, 63-66.

Buechley, R. W., Key, C. R., Morria, D. L., Morton, W. E., & Morgan, M. V. (1979). Altitude and ischemic heart disease in tricultural New Mexico: An example of confounding. *American Journal of Epidemiology, 109*, 663-666.

Bullough, B. (1972). Poverty, ethnic identity and preventive health care. *Journal of Health and Social Behavior, 13*, 347-359.

Bureau of Vital Statistics, Texas Department of Health (1981). *Vital statistics for Texas.* Austin: Texas Department of Health.

Caetano, R. (1983). Drinking patterns and alcohol problems among Hispanics in the U.S.: A review. *Drug and Alcohol Dependence, 18*, 1-15.

California Center for Health Statistics. (1983). *Diabetes among California Hispanics 1979-1980.* Data matters topical reports Nos. 83-05079.

Castro, F. G., Baezconde-Garbanati, L., & Beltran, H. (1985). Risk factors for coronary heart disease in Hispanic populations: A review. *Hispanic Journal of Behavioral Sciences, 7*, 153-175.

Christensen, B. L., Stallones, R. A., Insell, W., Jr., Gotto, A. M., & Taunton, D. (1981). Cardiovascular risk factors in a tri-ethnic population: Houston, Texas, 1972-1975. *Journal of Chronic Disease, 34*, 105-118.

Clark, M. (1959). *Health in the Mexican American culture.* Berkeley: University of California Press.

Devor, E. J., & Buechley, R. W. (1980). Gallbladder cancer in Hispanic New Mexicans. *Cancer, 45*, 1705-1712.

Eggers, P. W., Connerton, R., & McMullon, M. (1984). The Medicare experience with end-stage renal disease: Trends in incidence, prevalence, and survival. *Health Care Financing Review, 5*, 69-88.

206   *Aging and Health*

Ellis J. M. (1959). Mortality differentials for a Spanish-surname population group. *Southwestern Social Science Journal, 39*, 314-321.

Ellis, J. M. (1962). Spanish-surname mortality differences in San Antonio, Texas. *Journal of Health and Human Behavior, 3*, 125-127.

Estrada, L. F., Hernandez, J., & Alvirez, D. (1977). Using census data to study the Spanish heritage population of the United States. In C. H. Teller, L. F. Estrada, J. Hernandez, & D. Alvirez (Eds.), *Cuantos somos: A demographic study of the Mexican-American population* (pp. 13-59). Austin: Center for Mexican-American Studies.

Fillenbaum, G. (1979). Social context and self-assessment of health among the elderly. *Journal of Health and Social Behavior, 20*, 45-51.

Franco, L. J., Stern, M. P., Rosenthal, M., Haffner, S. M., Hazuda, H. P., & Convaux, P. J. (1985). Prevalence, detection, and control of hypertension in a biethnic community: The San Antonio Heart Study. *American Journal of Epidemiology, 121*, 684-696.

Frerichs, R. R., Chapman, J. M., & Maes, E. F. (1984). Mortality due to all causes and to cardiovascular diseases among seven race-ethnic populations in Los Angeles County, 1980. *International Journal of Epidemiology, 13*, 291-298.

Friis, R., Nanjundappa, G., Pendergast, T. J., & Welsh, M. (September-October, 1981). Coronary heart disease mortality and risk among Hispanics and non-Hispanics in Orange County, California. *Public Health Reports, 96*, 418-422.

Gardner, L. I., Stern, M. P., Haffner, S. M., Gaskill, S. P., Hazuda, H. P., Relethford, J. H., & Eifler, C. W. (1984). Prevalence of diabetes in Mexican Americans: Relationship to percent of gene pool derived from Native American sources. *Diabetes, 33*, 86-92.

Gilbert, M. J., & Cervantes, R. C. (1986). Patterns and practices of alcohol use among Mexican Americans: A comprehensive review. *Hispanic Journal of Behavioral Sciences, 8*, 1-60.

Gillespie, F. P., & Sullivan, T. A. (1983, April). What do current estimates of Hispanic mortality really tell us? Paper presented at the annual meeting of the Population Association of America, Pittsburgh.

Haber, R. J. (1985). Should postmenopausal women be given estrogen? Medical Staff Conference, University of California, San Francisco. *Western Journal of Medicine, 142*, 672-677.

Haffner, S. (1987). Hyperinsulinemia as a possible etiology for the high prevalence of non-insulin dependent diabetes in Mexican Americans. *Diabetes and Metabolism, 13*, 337-344.

Haffner, S., Stern, M., Hazuda, H., Pugh, J., & Patterson, J. (1987). Do upper-body and centralized adiposity measure different aspects of regional body-fat distribution? *Diabetes, 36*, 43-51.

Haffner, S., Stern, M., Hazuda, H., Rosenthal, M., Knapp, J., & Malina, R. (1986). Role of obesity and fat distribution in non-insulin-dependent diabetes mellitus in Mexican Americans and non-Hispanic Whites. *Diabetes Care, 9*, 153-161.

Hanis, C., Ferrell, R. E., & Schull, W. J. (1985). Hypertension and sources of blood pressure variability among Mexican Americans in Starr County, Texas. *International Journal of Epidemiology, 14*, 231-238.

Hanis, C., Ferrell, R. E., Barton, S. A., Aguilar, L., Garza-Ibarra, A., Tulloch, B. R., Garcia, C. A., & Schull, W. J. (1983). Diabetes among Mexican Americans in Starr County, Texas. *American Journal of Epidemiology, 118*, 659-672.

Hays-Bautista, D. E. (1980). Identifying "Hispanic" populations: The influence of research methodology upon public policy. *American Journal of Public Health, 70,* 353-356.

Hazuda, H. P., Stern, M. P., Gaskill, S. P., Haffner, S. M., & Gardner, L. I. (1983). Ethnic differences in health knowledge and behaviors related to the prevention and treatment of coronary heart disease: The San Antonio Heart Study. *American Journal of Epidemiology, 117,* 717-728.

Hernandez, J., Estrada, L., & Alvirez, D. (1973). Census data and the problem of conceptually defining the Mexican American population. *Social Science Quarterly, 53,* 671-687.

Hoppe, S. K., & Heller, P. L. (1975). Alienation, familism and the utilization of health services by Mexican Americans. *Journal of Health and Social Behavior, 16,* 304-314.

Kautz, J. A. (1982). Ethnic diversity in cardiovascular mortality. *Arteriosclerosis Reviews, 9,* 85-108.

Kautz, J. A., Bradshaw, B. S., & Fonner, E. (1981). Trends in cardiovascular mortality in Spanish-surnamed, other white, and black persons in Texas, 1970-1975. *Circulation, 64,* 730-735.

Kreiger, N., Kelsey, J., Holford, T., & O'Connor, T. (1982). An epidemiologic study of hip fracture in postmenopausal women. *American Journal of Epidemiology, 116,* 141-148.

Lee, E. S., Roberts, R. E., & Labarthe, D. R. (1976). Excess and deficit lung cancer mortality in three ethnic groups in Texas. *Cancer, 38,* 2551-2556.

Lopez-Aqueres, W., Kemp, B., Plopper, M., Staples, F. R., & Brummel-Smith, K. (1984). Health needs of the Hispanic elderly. *Journal of the American Geriatrics Society, 32,* 191-198.

MacMahon, B., Cole, P., Lin, T. M., Lowe, C. R., Mirra, A. P., Ravnihar, B., Salber, E. J., Valaoras, V. G., & Wuasa, S. (1970). Age at first birth and cancer of the breast: A summary of an international study. *WHO Bulletin, 43,* 209-221.

McDonald, E. J., & Heinze, E. B. (1978). *Epidemiology of cancer in Texas.* New York: Raven Press.

Maddox, G. L., & Douglass, E. B. (1973). Self-assessment of health: A longitudinal study of elderly subjects. *Journal of Health and Social Behavior, 14,* 87-93.

Madsen, W. (1964). *Mexican Americans of South Texas.* New York: Holt, Rinehart & Winston.

Manton, K. G., Poss, S. S., & Wing, S. (1979). The black/white crossover: Investigation from the perspective of the components of aging. *The Gerontologist, 19,* 291-300.

Marcus, A. C., & Crane, L. A. (1985). Smoking behavior among Latinos: An emerging challenge for public health. *American Journal of Public Health, 75,* 169-172.

Markides, K. S. (1983). Minority aging. In M. W. Riley, B. B. Hess & W. P. Frisbie (Eds.), *Aging in society: Selected reviews of recent research* (pp. 115-138). Hillsdale, NJ: Lawrence Erlbaum.

Markides, K. S., & Coreil, J. (1986). The health of Hispanics in the southwestern United States: An epidemiologic paradox. *Public Health Reports, 101,* 253-265.

Markides, K. S., & Coreil, J., & Ray, L. A. (1987). Smoking among Mexican Americans: A three-generations study. *American Journal of Public Health, 77,* 708-711.

Markides, K. S., Krause, N., & Mendes de Leon, C. (1988). Alcohol consumption among Mexican Americans: A three-generations study. *American Journal of Public Health, 78,* 1178-1181.

Markides, K. S., & Martin, H. W. (1979). Predicting self-rated health among the elderly. *Research on Aging, 1*, 97-112.

Markides, K. S., Martin, H. W., with Gomez, E. (1983). *Older Mexican Americans: A study in an urban barrio*. Monograph of the Center for Mexican American Studies. Austin: University of Texas Press.

Menck, H. R., Henderson, B. E., Pike, M. C., Mack, T., Martin, S. T., & Soottoo, J. (1975). Cancer incidence in the Mexican American. *Journal of the National Cancer Institute, 55*, 531-536.

Morris, D. L., Buechley, R. W., Key, C. R., & Morgan, M. V. (1978). Gallbladder disease and gallbladder cancer among American Indians in tricultural New Mexico. *Cancer, 42*, 2472-2477.

Moy, C. S., & Wilder, C. S. (1978). Health characteristics of minority groups, United States, 1976. Advance data from *Vital and Health Statistics*, Public Health Service (No. 27). Washington, DC: U.S. Government Printing Office.

Mullin, K., & Anderson, K. (1988). Cancer mortality in Illinois Mexican and Puerto Rican immigrants, 1979-1984. *International Journal of Cancer, 41*, 670-676.

National Center for Health Statistics. (1974). *Summary report: Final mortality statistics, 1970* (Vol. 22, No. 11). Rockville, MD: Public Health Service.

National Center for Health Statistics (1977). *Blood pressure levels of persons 6-74 years. United States 1971-1974* (National Health Survey, Series 11, No. 207). Hyattsville, MD: Author.

National Center for Health Statistics (1978). *Total serum cholesterol levels of adults 18-74 years: United States, 1971-1974* (National Health Survey, Series 11, No. 205). Hyattsville, MD: Author.

National Center for Health Statistics (1980a). *Health practices among adults: United States, 1977* (No. 64, DHHS Publication No. 81-1250). Hyattsville, MD: Public Health Service.

National Center for Health Statistics (1980b). *Health United States—1979*. Public Health Service. Washington, DC: U.S. Government Printing Office.

National Center for Health Statistics. (1984). *Health indicators for Hispanic, black, and white Americans. Vital Health Statistics*. ([10] No. 148). Washington, DC: U.S. Government Printing Office.

Newell, G. R., & Boutwell, W. B. (1981). Cancer differences among Texas groups: An hypothesis. *The Cancer Bulletin, 33*(3), 113-114.

Newell, G. R., & Mills, P. K. (1987). Low cancer rates in Hispanic women related to social and economic factors. *Women and Health, 11*, 23-35.

Newton, F. (1980). Issues in research and service delivery among Mexican American elderly. *The Gerontologist, 20*, 208-213.

Peters, P. K., Thomas, D., Hagan, D. G., Mack, T. M., & Henderson, B. E. (1986). Risk factors for invasive cervical cancer among Latinas and non-Latinas in Los Angeles County. *Journal of the National Cancer Institute, 77*, 1063-1077.

Pugh, J., Stern. M., Haffner, S., Eifler, C., & Zapata, M. (1988). Excess incidence of treatment of end-stage renal disease in Mexican Americans. *American Journal of Epidemiology, 127*, 135-144.

Relethford, J. H., Stern, M. P., Gaskill, S. P., & Hazuda, H. P. (1983). Social class, admixture, and skin color variation in Mexican Americans and Anglo-Americans living in San Antonio, Texas, with special reference to diabetes prevalence. *American Journal of Physical Anthropology, 61*, 97-102.

Research Group for Population-Based Cancer Registration. (1976). Cancer registries in Japan: Activities and incidence data. *Annual report of the Center for Adult Diseases* (Vol. 16, pp. 12-31). Osaka, Japan: Center for Adult Diseases.

Roberts, R. E. (1977). The study of mortality in the Mexican-American population. In C. H. Teller, L. F. Estrada, J. Hernandez, & D. Alvirez (Eds.), *Cuantos somos: A demographic study of the Mexican-American population* (pp. 131-155). Austin, TX: Center for Mexican American Studies.

Roberts, R. E., & Askew, C. (1972). A consideration of mortality in three subcultures. *Health Services Reports, 87*, 262-272.

Rosenwaike, I. (1988). Cancer mortality among Mexican immigrants in the United States. *Public Health Reports, 103*, 195-201.

Rotkin, I. D. (1973). A comparison review of key epidemiological studies in cervical cancer related to current searches for transmissible agents. *Cancer Research, 33*, 1353-1367.

Rubel, A. (1966). *Across the tracks: Mexican Americans in a Texas city.* Austin: University of Texas Press.

Samet, J. M., Key, C. R., Kutvirt, D. M., & Wiggins, C. L. (1980). Respiratory disease mortality in New Mexico's American Indians and Hispanics. *American Journal of Public Health, 70*, 492-497.

Samet, J. M., Schrag, S. D., Howard, C. A., Key, C. R., & Pathak, D. R. (1982). Respiratory disease in a New Mexico population sample of Hispanic and non-Hispanic whites. *American Review of Respiratory Diseases, 125*, 152-157.

Samet, J. M., Wiggins, C. L., Key, C. R., & Becker, C. R. (1988). Mortality from lung cancer and chronic obstructive pulmonary disease in New Mexico, 1958-82. *American Journal of Public Health, 78*, 1182-1186.

Saunders, L. (1954). *Cultural differences in medical care: The case of the Spanish-Speaking people of the Southwest.* New York: Russell Sage.

Savitz, D. A. (1986). Changes in Spanish-surname cancer rates relative to other whites, Denver area, 1969-71 to 1979-81. *American Journal of Public Health, 76*, 1210-1215.

Schoen, R., & Nelson, V. F. (1981). Mortality by cause among Spanish-surnamed Californians, 1969-1971. *Social Science Quarterly, 62*, 259-274.

Shai, D., & Rosenwaike, I. (1987). Mortality among Hispanics in metropolitan Chicago: An examination based on vital statistics data. *Journal of Chronic Diseases, (40)*, 445-451.

Shanas, E., & Maddox, G. L. (1976). Aging, health and the organization of health resources. In R. H. Binstock & E. Shanas (Eds.), *Handbook of the aging and the social sciences* (pp. 592-618). New York: Van Nostrand Reinhold.

Siegel, J. S., & Passel, J. (1979). Coverage of the Hispanic population of the United States in the 1970 census. *Current Population Reports* (Series P-23, No. 82). Washington, DC: U.S. Bureau of the Census.

Sievers, M., & Fisher, J. R. (1983). Cancer in North American Indians: Environment versus heredity. *American Journal of Public Health, 73*, 485-487.

State of New Mexico. (1980). *Unpublished raw data.* Santa Fe: New Mexico State Department of Health.

Stern, M. P., Bradshaw, B. S., Eifler, C. W., Fong, D. S., Hazuda, H. P., & Rosenthal, M. (1987). Secular decline in death rates due to ischemic heart disease in Mexican Americans and non-Hispanic whites in Texas, 1970-1980. *Circulation, 76*, 1245-1250.

Stern, M. P., & Gaskill, S. P. (1978). Secular trends in ischemic heart disease mortality from 1970 to 1976 in Spanish-surnamed and other white individuals in Bexar County, Texas. *Circulation, 58*, 537-543.

Stern, M. P., Gaskill, S. P., Allen, C. R., Jr., Garza, V., Gonzales, J. L., & Waldrop, R. H. (1981). Cardiovascular risk factors in Mexican Americans in Laredo, Texas. I. Prevalence of overweight and diabetes and distributions of serum lipids. II. Prevalence and control of hypertension. *American Journal of Epidemiology, 113*, 546-555, 556-562.

Stern, M. P., Gaskill, S. P., Hazuda, H. P., Gardner, L. I., & Haffner, S. M. (1983). Does obesity explain excess prevalence of diabetes among Mexican Americans? Results of the San Antonio Heart Study. *Diabetologia, 24*, 272-277.

Stern, M. P., Haskell, W. L., Wood, P. D., Osarin, K. E., King, A. B., & Farquhar, J. W. (1974). Affluence and cardiovascular risk factors in Mexican Americans and other whites in three northern California communities. *Journal of Chronological Disease, 28*, 623-636.

Sullivan, T. A., Gillespie, F. P., Hout, M., & Rogers, R. G. (1984). Alternative estimates of Mexican American mortality in Texas, 1980. *Social Science Quarterly, 65*, 609-617.

Terris, M., Wilson, F., Smith, H., Strung, E., & Nelson, J. H., Jr. (1967). Epidemiology of cancer of the cervix. V. The relationship of coitus to carcinoma of the cervix. *American Journal of Public Health, 57*, 840-847.

Thomas, D. B. (1979). Epidemiologic studies of cancer in minority groups in the United States. *National Cancer Institute Monograph, 53*, 103-113.

Trevino, K. M. (1982). Vital and health statistics for the U.S. Hispanic population. *American Journal of Public Health, 70*, 979-982.

Vernon, S. W., Tilley, B. C., Neale, A. V., & Steinfeldt, L. (1985). Ethnicity, survival, and delay in seeking treatment for symptoms of breast cancer. *Cancer, 55*, 1563-1571.

Weaver, J. L. (1973). Mexican-American health care behavior: A critical review of the literature. *Social Science Quarterly, 54*, 86-102.

West, K. M. (1978). *Epidemiology of diabetes and its vascular lesions.* New York: Elsevier.

Young, J. L. (1982). Cancer in minorities. In D. L. Parron, F. Solomon, & C. D. Jenkins (Eds.), *Behavior, health risks, and social disadvantage* (pp. 19-31). Washington, DC: National Academy Press.

Young, J. L., Percy, C. L., & Adire, A. J. (Eds.). (1981). Surveillance, epidemiology, and end results: Incidence and mortality data, 1973-1977. *National Cancer Institute Monograph, 57*, 1087.

CHAPTER 6

Aging and Health Among Navajo Indians

STEPHEN J. KUNITZ
JERROLD E. LEVY

INTRODUCTION

An extraordinary amount has been written about the culture, social organization, economic and demographic history, and health conditions of the Navajos. We shall merely summarize some of that material in this chapter, emphasizing those points that have particular bearing on our subject and referring the interested reader to the sources we shall cite for more detail.

In 1886, the Navajos signed a treaty that, among other things, provided for a reservation of some half million acres straddling the border between Arizona and New Mexico. Between 1880 and 1934, 14 Executive Orders expanded the reservation until, today, it covers about 24,000 square miles, mainly in northeastern and north central Arizona, but with significant land in northwestern New Mexico, and southeastern and south central Utah. The entire reservation is on the Colorado Plateau, a region characterized by relatively little rainfall except at higher elevations, the drainages of which flow into the San Juan, Colorado, and Little Colorado Rivers. Most of the reservation is in the Upper and Lower Sonoran life zones with vegetation ranging from pinon-juniper and sage brush to desert grassland and scrub. In the

AUTHORS' NOTE: Much of the work reported in this chapter was supported by grant R01 AG03403 from the National Institute on Aging.

mountains of northeastern Arizona, however, the Canadian and Transition life zones are found, in which Ponderosa pine and Douglas fir are common (Goodman, 1982).

Mineral resources underlying the reservation include coal, oil, uranium, and copper, most of it found in the eastern end where much extraction has occurred since the 1920s (Kelly, 1968; Parman, 1976). A large coalfield on Black Mesa in the central portion of the reservation has been strip-mined since the 1970s. Uranium was mined in the west but is no longer. The same is true of copper.

Although the reservation is bordered by the San Juan and Colorado rivers on the north and west, and cut by the Little Colorado River in the southwest, relatively little of the water has been available to the Navajos for agricultural or industrial purposes (Reno, 1981). Since the early ninteenth century, stock-raising rather than farming has been the Navajos' major source of livelihood in all but a very few areas of the reservation. As the population and livestock holdings increased more rapidly than new lands could be acquired, the reservation has been seriously overgrazed since the 1930s. A greater concentration of natural resources on and adjacent to the eastern portion of the reservation accounts for that area's denser population as well as for a large number of border towns and non-Indians.

The richness of mineral resources notwithstanding, the Navajo economy is underdeveloped. The lack of capital, the paucity of agricultural possibilities, bureaucratic impediments, and federal policies have combined to create what has been called a dual economy (Levy, 1980; Reno, 1981; for a slightly different view, see Wood, 1980). Heavily capitalized non-Navajo enterprises have dominated the extraction of nonrenewable resources without providing significant employment for Navajos. The largest proportion of tax revenues derived from these activities flow into state rather than tribal coffers, and the product is sold off the reservation for the benefit of distant, non-Indian communities. The isolation of the reservation and the unskilled labor force have discouraged business from locating on the reservation, and, to date, the only successful tribal enterprise is the harvesting of forest products.

With few opportunities for employment, and agriculture and stock-raising relatively unproductive, the Navajo economy is kept afloat by employment in federal, tribal, and state agencies providing health and human services, by several forms of welfare support, and by off-reservation wage work (Kunitz, 1983). In this context, the traditional extended family has continued to be adaptive as manpower must be deployed not only to accomplish many necessary domestic chores, such as sheepherding and hauling wood and water, but also to take advantage of whatever form of employment occasionally becomes available. The large, matrifocal, extended family shares vehicles and income derived from a variety of sources including various forms of welfare (Aberle, 1981; Henderson, 1979).

Differences in the availability of natural resources and access to border towns are reflected in regional differences in wage work, income, education levels, and dependence on welfare across the reservation. In general, the eastern end is characterized by greater involvement in the wage economy and the western end by greater dependence upon welfare (Kunitz, 1983). Demographically, too, there are significant differences. Population growth has been more rapid in the east than the west, despite the fact that mortality rates tend to be higher in the former than in the latter area. Fertility does not show such clear regional differences as it once did. In general, it appears that more rapid population growth in the east is due to immigration for sources of wage work.

Despite more rapid growth in the east than the west, it does not seem that the age structure of the population differs dramatically, at least at the level of land management districts (administrative units that ranged in size in 1980 from about 5,000 to over 20,000 people). So far as we have been able to estimate from the 1980 census, in which a considerable amount of underreporting seems to have occurred, the age distribution in all districts is approximately as follows: 0-18 years, 50 percent; 19-64 years, 45 percent; and 65 and above, 5 percent. At the community level, however, there are differences: in general, wage work settlements have younger populations than rural areas.

DEMOGRAPHY

The size and remoteness of the Navajo Reservation have made the population notoriously difficult to enumerate. Language barriers and lack of adequate records have made reporting of age at least as difficult. Both problems have been a source of frustration for researchers and bureaucrats alike for decades. Considering the difficulties, it is remarkable that there has been a good deal of consistency in estimates of the proportion of the Navajo population 65 years of age and above over the past 70 to 80 years. Table 6.1 displays population counts from several

Table 6.1 Navajo Population 65 and Above, 1910-1980

Year	Males ≥65	Males Total	Males %	Females ≥65	Females Total	Females %	Total Population ≥65	Total Population Total	Total Population %	Source
1910	437	11,305	3.8	466	11,072	4.2	903	23,377	4.0	Johnston 1966; 156
1930	593	19,746	3.0	579	19,280	3.0	1,172	39,026	3.0	Johnston 1966; 159
1945	1,220	30,897	3.9	976	30,165	3.2	2,196	61,062	3.6	Johnston 1966; 161
1957	1,781	40,638	4.4	1,613	41,062	3.9	3,394	81,700	4.2	Johnston 1966; 163
1961							2,912	93,377	3.1	Johnston 1966; 166
1972	2,863	66,244	4.3	2,604	69,608	3.7	4,838	135,852	3.6	BIA 1972 Carr 1978
1975	2,111			2,131			4,242			
1978	3,055	68,626	4.5	2,970	74,035	4.0	6,025	142,035	4.5	Navajo Tribe 1978
1980							4,553	129,868	3.5	Bureau of the Census 1980
							6,354		4.8	(adjusted for suppression)
							7,300			(adjusted for 15% underenumeration)

sources from 1910 through 1980. Despite undoubted inaccuracies, it is noteworthy that all of them place the proportion 65 and above at between 3.0 and 4.5 percent. By way of contrast, the proportion 65 and above in the entire U.S. population was 11.3 percent in 1980.

Although the population has grown rapidly during the course of this century, there is no evidence that the age structure has changed dramatically. The Navajos are still a young population. Fertility seems to have been high until the post-World War II years, at which time it began a slow decline from more than 40 to considerably less than 30 per 1,000 at present. At the same time, however, infant mortality began a very steep decline from about 140 to 17 per 1,000 live births. Declining infant and child mortality balanced declining fertility so that the overall impact was of continuing rapid population growth and a broad-based age pyramid. In future, as fertility continues to fall more rapidly than mortality, the age structure will gradually be transformed into one more nearly resembling that of the general U.S. population (Broudy & May, 1983). Of course, the number of people 65 and above has increased, though estimates of how many there are in this age group vary widely even from 1972 through 1980. Nonetheless, it is safe to assert that changes in the perceived or actual conditions of the elderly are unlikely to be due to a major change in age structure over the past 70 years.

MORTALITY

Not only has infant mortality declined, but the crude mortality rate for the entire population has as well, from perhaps 10-11 per 1,000 in 1945 to 6-7 per 1,000 at present (Kunitz, 1983). There is no evidence, however, that mortality among those 65 and above has changed very dramatically, though it must be emphasized that the data are not entirely adequate. The U.S. Public Health Service (1957) estimated that in the period 1949-1953, average annual age specific mortality of Navajos 65 and above was 30.6 per 1,000 in the population on the Arizona portion of the reservation (including a very small proportion of Hopis); 37.6 in the New Mexico Navajo population; and 50 in the Utah Navajo population. We have estimated below that the average annual age specific rate in 1972-1978 lies between 34 and 48 per 1,000 people 65 and above. Considering the difficulties of data collection and enumeration, the differences are not very impressive.

In order to estimate range of mortality rates for 1972-1978, we used as the numerator the deaths of all Indians 65 and above giving a reservation address during the period 1972-1978 (see Kunitz, 1983, for details). Since the denominator (all Navajos 65 and above living on reservation) was not accurately known, high and low estimates were used. The Navajo tribe's Department on Aging estimated the 1975 population to have been 4,242. Another tribal estimate, for 1978, was 6,025 people 65 and above (see Table 6.1). We have taken 6,000 as the upper boundary of the 1975 population. This upper limit may not be too far off the mark. The lower limit is almost certainly too low. The number of Navajos 65 and above enumerated on the reservation in the 1980 Census was 6,354. Based on our sampling in districts 1 and 3 on the western end of the reservation, we believe the census may have underenumerated the elderly population by as much as 15 percent. Nonetheless, for our purpose the range we have selected is adequate.

In Table 6.2 we have applied age-specific death rates for the entire U.S. population to the two estimates of the Navajo population in five-year segments starting at age 65. (The number of people in each age group was based on the proportions estimated by Carr [1978].) We have also displayed the observed number of deaths and the expected number per year based on the national figures. Notice that even using the extremely low population estimate of 4,000, the observed number of deaths is not significantly different from the expected in any age group.

The population data are far from adequate, and the mortality data may be also underreported to an unknown but not extravagant degree. Nonetheless, the evidence is reasonably good that mortality rates among elderly Navajos are no higher than the rates among non-Indians of the same age, and almost certainly are lower. Since mortality at younger ages is higher among Navajos than non-Navajos (Kunitz, 1983), this is an instance of the mortality "crossover," which has been observed among black Americans as well as in cross-national studies (Weatherby, Nan, & Isaac, 1983; Wing, Manton, Stallard, Hames, & Tyroler, 1985). Whether the crossover phenomenon is real or simply the result of bad data has been a matter of debate (Coale & Kisker, 1986). In a prospective field study among black Americans, it seems to have been confirmed. We believe it exists among Navajos, too, though at younger ages than among blacks.

Mortality "crossover" refers to the observation that, among certain populations, age-specific mortality is high at young and adult ages and relatively low at old age when compared to mortality rates in some

Table 6.2 Observed and Expected Deaths of Navajos ≥65, 1972-1978

Age	No. Navajo Deaths 1972-1978	Average per Year	1976 U.S. Death Rate per 1,000	Low Pop. Estimate	Expected Deaths per Year Based on Low Pop. Estimate*	High Pop. Estimate	Expected Deaths per Year Based on High Pop. Estimate**
65-69	291	42	25.4	1775	45	2664	68
70-74	269	38	39.5	945	37	1416	56
75-79	260	37	61.9	588	36	882	55
80-84	210	30	90.3	342	31	516	47
≥85	420	60	154.9	348	54	522	81

SOURCE: U.S. Dept. H.E.W., 1978.
*Population estimate of 4,000 Navajos ≥ 65 in 1975.
**Population estimate of 6,000 Navajos ≥ 65 in 1975.

standard, usually relatively affluent, populations. If one assumes that biological life span does not differ significantly among races or cross-nationally, then mortality must rise at some age among populations in which it has been low through most of life. Generally, it is relatively poor populations that experience high mortality in the young and adult years, presumably because of their exposure to a harsh environment, inadequate nutrition, and lack of access to medical care.

It is often suggested that among the populations with high mortality at young ages and relatively low mortality at older ages, a selection process is at work such that those who survive into old age are an especially hardy lot. We shall return to this issue below, but we may observe here that a study of elderly Indians and non-Indians (NICOA, 1981) found that self-reported functional impairment was greater among the former than the latter. And a prospective study of active life expectancy of a sample of the elderly population of Massachusetts found that income was positively related to length of time free of disability (Katz et al., 1983). Thus, there is some reason to expect that among the poor who survive into old age, health status will not neces-sarily be better than among the nonpoor.

Causes of death among populations experiencing the mortality crossover differ from those observed in more affluent populations. The former tend to die of so-called exogenous causes (e.g. infectious dis-eases and accidents) whereas the latter tend to die of what are called endogenous causes (e.g., cardiovascular diseases and cancers). These terms are not ideal since they assume a causal explanation, which, in the case of the so-called endogenous causes, must yet be demonstrated.

These patterns are observed among the Navajo. Carr and Lee (1978) estimated that elimination of motor vehicle accidents would increase Navajo male life expectancy at birth 5.17 years, and elimination of all other accidents would add 3.13 years. In contrast, elimination of auto-mobile accidents would have added only 0.93 years at birth to the life of U.S. white males in 1969-1971. Conversely, the elimination of cardiovascular disease would add 10.46 years of life at birth for white males, but only 3.31 for Navajo males. Women manifest similar pat-terns, though they lose fewer years of life as a result of accidents than do men.

Similar contrasts with the non-Navajo population emerge when we consider causes of death among the elderly (see Table 6.3). Heart diseases, malignant neoplasms, and cerebrovascular disease are all much higher among non-Navajos than even the highest estimated

Table 6.3 Leading Causes of Mortality of Navajos 65 and Above, Average Annual Rates/100,000 1972-78, Based on High and Low Population Estimates

Cause	Number	Low Rate*	High Rate**	U.S.A., 1976
Heart disease	242	576	864	2,393
Malignant neoplasms	174	414	621	979
Cerebrovascular disease	112	266	400	694
Accidents	150	357	535	104
Diabetes	33	78	117	108
Cirrhosis	12	28	43	36
Influenza/pneumonia	156	371	557	211
Arteriosclerosis	3	7	11	122
Total	1,450	3,452	5,178	5,429

*Based on 1975 population estimate of 6,000.
**Based on 1975 population estimate of 4,000.

Navajo rates, whereas the reverse is the case for accidents and influenza/ pneumonia.

Life expectancy of Navajo males is lower than that of females. Elsewhere we have suggested that a combination of forces has worked a change in the sex ratio of the reservation population from the 1940s to the present: declining maternal mortality, increasing male mortality from accidents, and differential rates of emigration seem to have resulted in a shift such that women now outnumber men (Kunitz & Slocumb, 1976). Though it is generally agreed that women outnumber men in the total population, there is disagreement as to whether the change has yet affected the oldest cohorts. Most figures suggest men still predominate at ages above 65, though Carr (1978) estimated 2,111 men and 2,131 women in 1975. The differences are not enormous, however, on the order of one to two percentage points: either 49 percent of men and 51 percent of women, or vice versa. If we say for the sake of simplicity that the numbers of men and women at 65 and over are esentially equal, we may calculate average annual age specific mortality rates for each sex. In the period 1972-1978, 806 men and 644 women died, giving a range of 38-54 per 1,000 for the former and 30-43 per 1,000 for the latter. Thus, there is some evidence that male and female mortality continue to differ in older age groups.

The implications in respect of the situation of elderly widows are important: projections of the growth of the elderly population based upon the assumption that current mortality trends will continue indicate that the proportion of men and women at 65 and above will have shifted from approximate equality to 43 percent of men and 57 percent of women by the year 2000 (Carr, 1978).

Many of these inferences from reservation-wide data are supported by data from a prospective study of the health status and mortality experience of a sample of 271 Navajo women and men from the western end of the reservation. They were interviewed during the twelve-month period September 1, 1982 to August 30, 1983. During that year and for the next three years, we followed their mortality experience. We used key informants, regular reviews of hospital records, and two reviews of death certificates in the State Health Department in Phoenix for ascertainment of death. The first death certificate review was done in April 1985, the second in August 1986. The last wave of interviews of key informants was in June 1986. We have no reason to believe that any deaths went undiscovered during that period. All people were considered to have been under observation

Table 6.4 Mortality by Age and Sex

Status at Time of Follow-up	Age at Time of Follow-up			
	< 75		≥ 75	
	Male	Female	Male	Female
Dead	8	0	14	15
Alive	40	56	62	75
chi-square	10.111		0.0888	
d.f.	1		1	
p value	<.01		>.05	

from the time of interview to the time of death or until June 30, 1986. The average number of months of observation was 37 per person.

Table 6.4 displays the age and sex distribution and vital status of the sample at the time of follow-up. There are two noteworthy results. First, significantly more men than women died below the age of 75. This is consistent with findings we shall describe in more detail below, that women in this age group reported lower scores than men on the Sickness Impact Profile, a measure of functional status, as well as lower rates of hospital use. Second, there is no significant difference between the sexes at ages 75 and above.

Thirty-seven people died during the period of observation, giving an average annual rate of about 45 per 1,000, which is close to the top of the range we have estimated for the entire Navajo population 65 years of age and above. When we applied the age-specific death rates for the entire U.S. population (see Table 6.2) to the same five-year age intervals of the people in our sample, we noted that the total expected number of deaths (about 50) was higher than the observed number (37), and that the same was true in each age group.

There are several questions raised by the low mortality of elderly Navajos. First, do either one or both sexes account for the effect? Second, what causes of death characterize this low mortality population? And third, does high mortality at younger ages result in selection of an especially healthy older population?

In respect to the first question, Table 6.5 displays observed and expected deaths in each age-sex category based on rates in the total U.S. population. Though the numbers are small, the evidence suggests that the crossover begins later for men than women.

Table 6.5 Observed and Expected Navajo Deaths by Age and Sex (Western Navajo Sample)

Sex	Age	U.S. Pop., 1976 Death Rate 1000	No. Navajos in 1982	Expected Deaths in 3 Yrs.	Observed (age at time of interview)
Men	65-9	35.9 ⎫ 45.1	71	9-10	10
	70-4	54.3 ⎭			
	75-9	82.6 ⎫			
	80-4	115.2 ⎬ 125.8	53	20	12
	85+	179.8 ⎭			
Women	65-9	17.1 ⎫ 22.8	83	6	2
	70-4	28.6 ⎭			
	75-9	17.1 ⎫			
	80-4	76.3 ⎬ 89.3	64	17	13
	85+	143.1 ⎭			

In respect to causes, as mortality rates decline and chronic, noninfectious diseases become more significant than infectious disease, it becomes increasingly difficult to determine a single cause of death. Generally, multiple contributing causes are involved, particularly among elderly people. The problem is exacerbated in our sample, among whom 11 (30 percent) died at home without significant investigation of the circumstances. In Table 6.6 we display the causes of death of the people in our sample as extracted from medical records and death certificates. No autopsies were done.

The cases diagnosed as heart failure (3), tuberculosis (1), natural causes (2), and cardiac arrest (1) all died at home and were investigated by a police coroner. Only one of them, a 91-year-old woman, had been in hospital during the period 1980-1983, and she had been diagnosed then as having ischemic heart disease. The 66-year-old man who died of a presumed cardiac arrest had a history of chronic alcohol abuse and had a chronic subdural hematoma and cerebral atrophy. He was found dead in the shower. One of the men with heart failure was 65 at the time of interview, in remarkably good health, and died while herding sheep. The 82-year-old woman diagnosed as having died from tuberculosis

Table 6.6 Causes of Death, 1983-1986

Heart Disease	
Acute myocardial infarction	5
"Heart failure"	3
Cardio-respiratory arrest	1
Cardiac arrest	1
Cerebrovascular accident	2
Respiratory	
Tuberculosis	1
Chronic obstructive pulmonary	2
Pneumonia	3
Genito-urinary	
Renal failure	3
Cancer	
Malignant mesothelioma	1
Accident	
Pedestrian struck by motor vehicle	3
Fall followed by subdural hematoma	1
Violence, exacerbating "debility"	1
Fall followed by fractured femur	1
Miscellaneous	
Unknown	5
"Natural causes"	2
Bubonic plague	1
Chronic comatose state and aspiration pneumonia	1

was found dead in bed and in the hospital record had no evidence of active disease. Thus, it is not clear how accurate many of these diagnoses are.

On the other hand, of the five cases of myocardial infarction, two were diagnosed in hospital and two died in cars while being transported to hospital and had histories compatible with myocardial infarction. The fifth died in a nursing home of aspiration pneumonia while in coma after an infarction. This person also had a history of ischemic heart disease and bouts of respiratory failure secondary to old tuberculosis. Likewise, the two cases attributed to respiratory failure had well-documented histories (one died in a nursing home, the other at home), as did the two cases who died of strokes (one in hospital, the other in a nursing home). Of the three cases of renal failure, two were clearly diabetic in origin while the third was of unknown etiology. This person had pneumonia as the immediate cause of death.

The man who was debilitated and had been badly beaten, probably by his alcoholic son, died in a nursing home. It is not certain that the beating contributed to his death, however, and it is with some reservations that we have listed it as due to violence. The 75-year-old man who died after a fall and fractured femur had been in hospital for treatment of esophageal dysmotility secondary to diabetes. He had also been very depressed.

We have given these examples to indicate the degree of certainty and uncertainty surrounding the labels we have applied. While observing due caution, we believe we may offer several observations based on these data. First, when compared to the causes of death observed among people 65 and above at Many Farms in the central part of the reservation 25 years ago, myocardial infarctions seem to be more frequent (five definite and five others probable) (Fulmer & Roberts, 1983). Second, auto accidents continue to be an important cause of death among men in this age group, as they are among younger men. Third, respiratory failure secondary to tuberculosis is a significant cause (either contributing or underlying) of death but will probably diminish since active tuberculosis has diminished very markedly over the last four decades. And fourth, renal failure caused by diabetes is a problem that will almost certainly become more significant since there is some evidence that the incidence of diabetes is increasing among Navajos as it is among many other Indian populations.

Cause of death among the elderly is related to the question of selection of especially fit people through the filter of high mortality among the young. The selection hypothesis would be particularly convincing if people died young of the same diseases that are important among the elderly. Thus, if the high rate of young adult mortality was accounted for by heart disease, and if no one with heart disease survived beyond age 65, then, of course, heart disease would not be a cause of death among the elderly. But it is accidents that account for the excess mortality of the young, not heart disease. One might argue that the people who die young of accidents include a disproportionate number who, had they lived, would have died of cardiovascular disease and cancer, the diseases of the elderly that seem to be rare among Navajos. But it is difficult to make a convincing case for this possibility in the absence of adequate data on the psychosocial and physiological characteristics of accident victims.

In addition, as we shall discuss in more detail below, rough measures of function indicate that health status of our sample of Navajos is not significantly different from that of a sample of the Massachusetts population of the same age. By these criteria, then, high mortality at young ages has not resulted in an especially fit older population.

Several considerations lead us to pursue the question further, however. First, measures of function seem to reflect two different processes: classifiable nosographic entities on one hand and nonspecific sequelae of aging on the other. Second, lower than expected numbers of deaths is surely a reflection of some element of health status. Third, among men under 75 who died were a few with very extensive hospitalizations. Indeed, they had spent significantly more days in hospital than controls. This was not the case for older women and men, among whom hospital use did not differ between those who died and those who did not. If extensiveness of hospital use is a valid reflection of severity of illness—as we believe it to be in these instances—then we do have some support for the notion that among young-old men mortality does exert a selective force. Before dealing further with this question, we turn to the issue of morbidity.

TREATED MORBIDITY

The number of Navajos 65 and above hospitalized each year has increased slowly since 1972; at the same time, average length of hospital stay has decreased very dramatically (Kunitz, 1983). Over the decade 1972-1982 the number of hospital discharges of elderly Navajos increased about 21 percent (from 1,431 to 1,735), whereas average length of stay declined about 44 percent (from 15.1 to 8.4 days). The impact on total patient days was substantial: a decline of about 33 percent.

The pattern is not unique to the elderly. During the 1970s total Navajo hospitalizations remained roughly constant, whereas average length of stay for all causes considered individually or together declined. Presumably, this was the result of a combination of factors: readier access to hospitals, improvements in health status, and Indian Health Service policies among them.

In Table 6.1 we have displayed estimates of the number of Navajos 65 and above living on reservation in 1980. A reasonable range is between 6,000 and 7,300. During the four fiscal years 1980-1983, there were 6,416 hospital discharges in this same population, or an average of 1,604 per year. The average annual discharge rate is thus between 219 and 267 per 1,000, considerably lower than the rate in the general U.S. population, which increased from 355 to 399 per 1,000 from 1977 to 1982 (Waldo & Lazenby, 1984, p. 7). Only with an excessively low estimate of 4,500 people 65 and above in the early 1980s would the Navajo rate have reached 356 per 1,000. Thus, there is reasonably good evidence that elderly Navajos use hospitals less than the rest of the population of the same age.

Table 6.7 displays primary discharge diagnoses of elderly Navajos as compared with the general population of the same age. Navajos have higher discharge rates for infective and parasitic diseases. For all other categories their rates are lower than, or the same as, those of the general population. Of the three most important categories for Navajos—diseases of the circulatory, respiratory, and digestive systems—the latter two occur at about the same rate as in the general population and the first occurs at a substantially lower rate. These diagnostic patterns are approximately what one would expect based on the distribution of causes of death. Circulatory diseases and neoplasms are less significant among Navajos than they are among the general population. Diseases of the respiratory system cover a wide assortment of infectious and noninfectious maladies. Among Navajos, influenza and pneumonia are especially important as a cause of both mortality and hospitalized morbidity. With the available data it is difficult to be certain how the non-Navajo hospital discharge pattern of respiratory diseases may differ.

It is clear that infectious diseases, while still significant among elderly Navajos, are no longer the leading cause of mortality and hospitalized morbidity. In respect of the latter, while respiratory diseases (primarily influenza and pneumonias of all sorts) are the single leading discharge diagnosis, circulatory diseases consume more hospital days. Indeed, average lengths of stay differ significantly among primary diagnostic categories (p .0001 by analysis of variance), and of the three most significant rubrics, respiratory diseases require shorter lengths of stay than the others (using Duncan's multiple range test). This is surprising considering that the average age of patients with respiratory diseases is significantly greater than that of patients with either digestive (mostly gall bladder) or circulatory diseases, 78.7 for the former vs. 76.7 for the latter two. In fact, neither age nor sex is related to length of stay (p 0.57 by analysis of covariance).

Table 6.7 Discharge Diagnoses, Navajos ≥ 65, 1980-1983 (F.Y.)

First Listed Discharge Diagnoses	No. Discharges	ALOS	Total # Days	Average Annual Rate/1,000 Low*	Average Annual Rate/1,000 High**	U.S. Rate/1,000 1982 (≥65)
Infective and parasitic	334	9.7	3,227	11.4	13.9	5
Neoplasms	423	10.9	4,600	14.5	17.6	42
Endocrine,etc.	270	8.8	2,385	9.2	11.3	16
Diseases of blood, etc.	56	9.9	552	1.9	2.3	6
Mental disorders	101	9.8	987	3.5	4.2	10
Diseases of the nervous system	478	6.4	3,043	16.4	19.9	28
Circulatory system	863	8.9	7,734	29.5	35.9	117
Respiratory system	1,005	6.9	6,948	34.4	41.9	37
Digestive system	827	7.8	6,474	28.3	34.4	50
Genitourinary system	579	7.7	4,460	19.8	24.1	28
Skin and subcutaneous tissue	161	13.2	2,124	5.5	6.7	5
Musculo-skeletal	118	10.3	1,211	4.0	4.9	22
Congenital anomalies	10	6.2	62	0.3	0.4	1.0
Symptoms, etc.	434	6.2	2,711	14.9	18.1	3.0
Accidents, etc.	522	9.2	4,801	17.9	21.8	28.0
Special conditions, tests, etc.	222	9.9	2,195	7.6	9.3	2.0

SOURCE: Waldo and Lazenby (1984:9).
*Low rate based upon population estimate of 7,300.
**High rate based upon population estimate of 6,000.

THE USE OF LONG TERM CARE

Unlike hospital use, which is provided free to all Native American beneficiaries of the Indian Health Service, the use of long-term care facilities is a morass of conflicting bureaucratic rules and regulations. Different states and agencies have different policies regarding payments for different levels of care. Lack of uniformity is reflected in the lack of any register that would allow one to find out how many elderly Navajos are in such facilities at any given time. Diligent searching in the spring of 1984 indicated that a total of 70 Navajos 65 years of age and above were in one or another of two extended care facilities on the reservation. Another 73 were in facilities in border towns, though one was as far away as Phoenix. The vast majority of off-reservation placements were in facilities in New Mexico and were either from the New Mexico part of the reservation or from adjacent parts of Arizona. Similarly, only 17 of 70 patients in reservation facilities were from the western end of the reservation (districts 1-8). The discrepancy is largely accounted for by more liberal policies in New Mexico and the location of reservation facilities in the east-central part of the reservation. There were only one patient from district 1 and three from district 3 in reservation extended care facilities. There was only one patient from either of these two districts in an off-reservation facility.

It is possible that a few elderly nursing home residents were missed, but it is unlikely that the number was large. If we assume generously that 15 to 20 were missed, and that the number of Navajos 65 and above on the reservation in 1984 was somewhere between 6,000 and 7,300, then the proportion in all levels of long-term care was between 2.1 and 2.6 percent.

The National Master Facility Inventory showed that in 1980 the proportion of Arizona residents 65 and above who were in nursing and related homes (not including hospital-based nursing homes and ECFs) was 2.7 percent. The proportion of institutionalized New Mexico residents of the same age was 2.4 percent. Considering all states, there was an almost perfect correlation ($r=.99$) between the proportion of state residents 65 and above in such facilities and the number of beds per 1,000 people 65 and above in each state (calculated from NMFI, 1983). These observations suggest, first, that Navajos do not differ dramatically from all elderly residents of Arizona and New Mexico in the degree to which they use long-term facilities, and, second, that the availability of beds is the major determinant of utilization. The fact that average length of hospital stay has declined significantly for Navajos in this age group since the early 1970s also indicates that these institutions are not being used as ECFs and nursing homes.

It is important to keep in mind that availability of beds seems to be the major limiting factor in utilization, for along with the lower mortality and hospital utilization rates among people 65 and above, this may be interpreted to mean that elderly Navajos are remarkably fit and not in need of services comparable to those of other elderly Americans. The results we shall report below suggest this is not necessarily the case.

SELF-REPORTED LEVEL OF FUNCTION

In this section we shall consider several measures of health status based on our study of 271 elderly Navajo men and women: medical diagnoses gleaned from informants' medical records; self-reported level of functioning based on standardized scales, the Sickness Impact Profile (SIP); hospital use immediately prior to and during the study period, January 1, 1980 to June 30, 1983; and the interrelations between and among them.

The SIP scales are of two sorts: (1) physical mobility and self care, and (2) psychosocial functioning. As the interviews were lengthy, we could not use all the scales included in the original instrument (Department of Health Services, 1977). Moreover, a few of the original questions in the scales we did use were inappropriate in the Navajo context and were dropped. Others had to be reworded: e.g., climbing stairs was changed to climbing hills. There are a number of ways that the scales have been scored in other studies (Gilson et al., 1975). We chose the simplest, summing the scores assigned by the developers of the scales (Bergner et al., 1976a; Bergner, Bobbitt, Pollard, Martin, & Gibson, 1976b; Pollard, Bobbitt, Bergner, Martin, & Gilson, 1976). We also scored them on an ordinal three-point scale: yes, sometimes, and no. The results are so highly correlated with the assigned interval scores that only the assigned scores were used throughout.

High scores on the Depression and SIP scales reflect many affirmative answers and indicate worse levels of self-reported functioning in the domain tapped by any particular scale. The first set, AMBSIP (ambulation), MOBSIP (mobility), and BCMSIP (body care and movement), are all highly intercorrelated among both men and women. They

Table 6.8 Means and Medians of SIP and Depression Scales

		Women <75	Men <75	Women ≥75	Men ≥75
PHYSIP	mean*	324	376	664	554
	median	216	283	544	380
ALBSIP	mean**	100	114	180	158
	median	78	78	142	78
SOISIP	mean***	86	99	146	150
	median	44	80	84	80
TOTSIP	mean*	511	593	958	856
	median	378	512	831	660
DEPRESS	mean***	5.4	3.6	4.3	3.5
	median	4.0	2.0	3.5	2.0

ANOVAs   *Kruskall-Wallis ANOVA*   all differences are significant
*p = .0001
**p = .0075
***p = .04

sum to a total score: PHYSIP. The second set, ALBSIP (alertness behavior) and SOISIP (social interaction), are also highly correlated for both men and women. All five scales sum to TOTSIP. The purpose of these scales is to assess levels of function as they relate to health status, not to make a diagnosis of a medically classifiable disease.

Table 6.8 displays the means and medians of the SIP and Depression scales for each age-sex group. The very large differences between these two measures, in some instances with the mean often being substantially higher than the median, indicate the presence of extreme values that may make the use of parametric statistical tests of questionable appropriateness. In some of the subsequent analyses, therefore, we have done nonparametric instead of, or in addition to, parametric analyses.

The most striking feature of the results is that, with one exception, the Depression scale, women below the age of 75 rank lowest on all the SIP scales. Men below age 75 are next lowest on the PHYSIP and TOTSIP scales, and men and women 75 and above are always higher on each scale than the two younger groups. The Alertness Behavior and Social Interaction scales differ from the others. With regard to the means, the two older groups have significantly higher scores than the younger ones. With regard to the medians of the Alertness Behavior scale, however, men and women below 75 and men 75 and above are

Table 6.9 Intercorrelations of SIP and Depression Scales

A. Women*	AMB SIP	MOB SIP	BCM SIP	SOI SIP	ALB SIP	PHY SIP	TOT SIP	DEP RESS
AMBSIP	—	.63	.70	.61	.36	.87	.79	.13
MOBSIP	.57	—	.68	.62	.44	.81	.78	.07
BCMSIP	.77	.74	—	.73	.55	.94	.92	.24
SOISIP	.32	.49	.50	—	.57	.75	.85	.29
ALBSIP	.51	.49	.57	.46	—	.53	.72	.44
PHYSIP	.89	.80	.96	.48	.59	—	.95	.19
TOTSIP	.80	.79	.91	.71	.75	.94	—	.31
DEPRESS	.20	.31	.25	.23	.29	.27	.31	—

*women < 75 below the diagonal; women ≥ 75 above the diagonal

women < 75
$r = .46$ $p = .0001$
$r = .21$ $p = .05$

women ≥ 75
$r = .49$ $p = .0001$
$r = .24$ $p = .05$

B. Men**	AMB SIP	MOB SIP	BCM SIP	SOI SIP	ALB SIP	PHY SIP	TOT SIP	DEP RESS
AMBSIP	—	.59	.77	.41	.48	.87	.81	.09
MOBSIP	.63	—	.71	.62	.51	.80	.82	.20
BCMSIP	.73	.45	—	.41	.44	.96	.86	.00
SOISIP	.34	.49	.22	—	.63	.49	.76	.09
ALBSIP	.30	.45	.26	.68	—	.51	.75	.21
PHYSIP	.90	.76	.93	.40	.40	—	.92	.00
TOTSIP	.81	.76	.84	.68	.69	.91	—	.07
DEPRESS	.11	.13	.14	.48	.47	.18	.35	—

**men < 75 below the diagonal; men ≥ 75 above the diagonal

men < 75
$r = .45$ $p = .001$
$r = .22$ $p = .05$

men ≥ 75
$r = .50$ $p = .0001$
$r = .27$ $p = .05$

the same while women 75 and above have substantially higher scores. With regard to Social Interaction, men and women 75 and above and men below 75 have indentical scores, while women below 75 have the lowest scores. Women below 75 clearly differ from women 75 and above by always reporting better levels of function. Men in each group tend to be more nearly the same, sometimes resembling the younger women and sometimes the older. Means are always higher than medians, sometimes very much so, indicating the presence of extreme cases. The smallest differences are found among men below 75.

Table 6.9 shows that within each age-sex group all the scales are highly correlated. We have displayed only Pearson's correlations, but rank order correlations give essentially identical results.

Table 6.10 Hospital Use 1980-83, by Age-Sex Group*

Hospitalized in 1980-83	Women < 75	Men < 75	Women ≥ 75	Men ≥ 75
Not hospitalized	64	43	35	32
Hospitalized	18	27	27	22

df = 3
X^2 = 9.29
p = 0.025
*unknowns omitted

The second set of measures of health status is made up of indicators of hospital utilization in 1980-1983: number of hospitalizations, total number of days in hospital, average length of hospital stay, and number of surgical procedures. There is no distinction made among tests with regard to complexity or cost. A barium enema and a blood count are given the same weight. This is for two reasons: (1) the review of all the charts was done by one person over a two-month period, and more refined weightings were not feasible in the limited time available; and (2) the Public Health Service does not charge for tests or other services (unless the patient has third party coverage) so there is no uniform and readily available way to review bills and use dollar amounts as a measure of the intensity of use of various services, including laboratories. Moreover, since some patients were treated elsewhere and only discharge summaries were available, there is inevitably under-counting of diagnostic tests. Finally, for simplicity and because out-patient services are obtained in a wide variety of clinics in the region, no effort was made to count outpatient laboratory work or visits.

Ninety-four people in our sample were hospitalized a total of 175 times between January 1, 1980, and June 30, 1983. Table 6.10 gives the distribution by age and sex. Considering their lower SIP scores, it is not surprising to discover that women below the age of 75 were hospital-ized significantly less than the other three age-sex groups.

The measures of hospital use are continuous variables, but since most of the people in our sample were not hospitalized during the years 1980-1983, it would be inappropriate to consider them all together when correlating, say, the SIP scales with measures of hospital use. What we have done, therefore, is, first, compare the people who were hospitalized with those who were not and, second, examine the people who were hospitalized in respect of their utilization patterns.

Table 6.11 Logistic Regression: Hospital Use in 1980-1983 Adjusted for Age, Sex, PHYSIP

Age		*Male*		*Female*	
		Low PHYSIP	*High PHYSIP*	*Low PHYSIP*	*High PHYSIP*
< 75		9/36	16/32	6/52	12/30
≥ 75		7/24	15/30	6/20	21/40

Parameter	*Estimate*	*S.E.*	*Odds Scale*	*95% Confidence Interval*
Age	.43	.27	1.53	(0.90, 2.64)
Sex	−.31	.27	0.73	(0.43,1.26)
PHYSIP	1.81	.27	6.11	(3.56, 10.49)

In Table 6.11 we have displayed the results of a logistic regression with age, sex, and PHYSIP as the independent variables, and hospitalization in 1980-1983 (yes/no) as the dependent variable. Age is not quite significant and PHYSIP is very significant. There is no association with sex. On the other hand, the same analysis with first ALBSIP and then SOISIP substituted for PHYSIP shows that only age is significantly associated with hospitalization. Thus, PHYSIP is most significantly related to hospital use, with age exerting a slight independent effect, which, however, becomes much stronger when PHYSIP is removed from the analysis. This, of course, is because most people with high PHYSIP scores are older than those with low scores.

Turning our attention to those who were hospitalized, notice first in Table 6.12 that measures of hospital use (number of days, tests, and admissions) are significantly correlated in each age-sex group. Second, only among men and women below 75 are there significant relationships between the SIP scores and the various measures of hospital use. Among people 75 and above there are no significant correlations.

To explain these patterns it is useful to consider our respondents more closely. Table 6.13 indicates that there is a significant difference between people younger than 75 and those 75 and above in respect to the number hospitalized for an extreme number of days (40 or more over the 3.5 years 1980-1983).

When we pick out the people in our sample with extreme PHYSIP scores (in the top 10 percent) and cross classify those who were hospitalized by age, hospital use, and PHYSIP, we obtain the results dis-

Table 6.12 Intercorrelations of Hospital and SIP Variables
(hospitalized respondents only)

A. Men*				*Pearson's r*		
	Days	*Tests*	*No. Hosp*	*PHYSIP*	*ALBSIP*	*SOISIP*
Days in hospital	—	.94	.87	.13	−.11	−.13
No. tests	.89	—	.78	.10	−.10	−.10
No. hospitalizations	.48	.35	—	.07	−.21	−.21
PHYSIP	.47	.31	.71	—	.43	.31
ALBSIP	.10	.05	.46	.35	—	.45
SOISIP	.26	.21	.29	.26	.74	—

*men < 75, below diagonal; men ≥ 75 above diagonal		Men < 75 r = .46 p = .01		Men ≥ 75 r = .51 p = .01		

B. Women**	*Days*	*Tests*	*No. Hosp*	*PHYSIP*	*ALBSIP*	*SOISIP*
Days in hospital	—	.83	.44	−.03	−.08	−.14
No. tests	.45	—	.49	−.21	−.13	−.22
No. hospitalizations	.36	.85	—	.01	.12	.09
PHYSIP	.25	.77	.59	—	.70	.80
ALBSIP	.28	.65	.60	.78	—	.80
SOISIP	.25	.75	.53	.92	.71	—

**women < 75, below diagonal; women ≥ 75 above diagonal		Women < 75 r = .45 p = .05		Women ≥ 75 r = .44 p = .02		

played in Table 6.14. Though the numbers in some of the cells are vanishingly small, it is striking nonetheless that people with high PHYSIP scores and low hospital use are almost invariably 75 years of age and above. Those few people with extreme numbers of hospital days are almost invariably below the age of 75, whether or not they have high PHYSIP scores.

The reasons for these patterns have to do with what the SIP scales measure on the one hand and with diagnostic patterns and hospital use on the other. As noted previously, the SIP scales measure self-reported level of functioning, not specific diseases. We may illustrate the differences by describing briefly the people in the various cells of Table 6.14.

Among the eight people hospitalized for 40 days or more were four women below the age of 75. One had had a severe stroke that left her disabled. She had spend much time in hospital and was interviewed at

Table 6.13 Number of Hospital Days by Age-Sex Group*

No. Day 1980-1983	Women < 75	Men < 75	Women ≥75	Men ≥75
40+ days	4	3	0	1
< 40 days	13	19	27	21

* unknown omitted
x^2 (< 75 vs. ≥ 75) = 4.86
d.f. = 1
p = .05

Table 6.14 Hospital Use and PHYSIP Scores by Age*

		< 75	≥ 75
A.	PHYSIP low, hosp. low	32	36
B.	PHYSIP high, hosp. low	1	12
C.	PHYSIP low, hosp. high	5	0
D.	PHYSIP high, hosp. high	2	1

A × B, chi-square = 5.4, p = .02
B × C, p = .005 (Fisher's exact test)
B × D, N.S.
(A+B) × (C+D), x^2 = 4.68, p ≈ .05
*Unknowns omitted

home shortly before being placed in a nursing home. Another woman in this group had a long history of alcohol abuse and had recently developed active tuberculosis. She was not disabled but had spent four months in hospital. Yet another had experienced several losses of near kin in the preceding several years and had subsequently gone into a severe depression, which was compounded by Parkinson's disease and an organic brain syndrome. She was living with kin and seemed to be stable when interviewed. The last person in this group had had tuberculosis, which had left her with little functioning lung, and she was in and out of the hospital with episodes of respiratory failure.

One of the three men below the age of 75 also had old tuberculosis and numerous episodes of respiratory failure. Like the woman described above, he required oxygen at home and was severely disabled. He also suffered from diabetes and hypertension. The second man in this age group with much time in hospital suffered from diabetes and chronic renal failure for which he required frequent dialysis. He also had lost both legs in an accident many years previously and was confined to a wheelchair. (Both these men died in the follow-up period.) The third had a long history of tuberculosis in addition to benign essential hypertension and diabetes. His lengthy hospitalization, however, was due to the development of peritonitis, which required rather extensive abdominal surgery. The only person above the age of 75 with 40 or more days in hospital was a man of 83 who had tuberculosis (old), diabetes, congestive heart failure, eczema, cellulitis, and urinary tract infections.

By way of contrast, consider the 13 people with high PHYSIP scores and less than 40 days of hospital use. Among them was one woman below 75 who was seriously disabled from an old hip fracture. In addition, she was diabetic, had mild congestive heart failure, and had suffered a pulmonary embolism. She had been hospitalized a total of 19 days. The other twelve were all 75 or older. Three had chronic brain syndrome; six had severe osteoarthritis; one had a combination of chronic brain syndrome and osteoarthritis; and two had Parkinson's disease.

Among the people with low PHYSIP scores and less than 40 days of hospital use were 32 below 75 and 36, 75 and above. In the former group were 20 men and 12 women. For ease of exposition we shall consider only those with more than 10 and less than 40 days of hospitalization. Nine men and four women below age 75 fell in this category. Among the men were two admitted with benign prostatic hypertrophy and four with pneumonia, one of whom also had had a subdural hematoma some years previously from which he still suffered symptoms, another of whom had chronic nephritis and rheumatoid arthritis, a third who had congestive heart failure, emphysema, and bronchiectasis, and the last with with diabetes and hypertension. A seventh man had an acute myocardial infarction; the eighth had gout, rheumatoid arthritis, and ankylosis of several joints; and the ninth had old tuberculous osteomyelitis requiring surgery and chemotherapy. Among the women was one with life-long grand mal epilepsy, who had fallen into a fire and been burned; another with gall bladder disease; a third with diarrhea, pyelonephritis, osteoarthritis, and panhypopituitarism (as a result of postpartum hemorrhage many years previously); and a fourth with diabetes, uterine prolapse, and a urinary tract infection.

Among the 36 people 75 and above who had been hospitalized less than 40 days were 14 men and 22 women. Seven of the former and 10 of the latter had been hospitalized more than 10 days. Three of the men had pneumonia, in addition to which one had old tuberculosis, another had gall bladder disease, and the last had diabetes. Another man had renal calculi and benign prostatic hypertrophy. The fifth had burns of the face and hand, the sixth had a fractured femur, and the seventh, with the greatest number of days (more than 30) was diagnosed simply as senile. Two of the women had pneumonia, in addition to which one had gall bladder disease and the other emphysema. A third had gall bladder disease and bubonic plague. Two had ischemic heart disease, two others had cholecystitis, another had diarrhea, and the last had hypertension, poorly defined cerebrovascular disease, diabetes, and diverticulitis.

This lengthy litany should help make clear why the correlations are significant for the men and women below the age of 75 but not for those who are older. Among the younger group are a few extreme cases, people who suffer from severe chronic diseases that require much time in hospital and also cause very substantial functional impairment. It is these extreme cases who make the correlations significant. Among the people 75 and above are many people with considerable loss of function, but the loss of function is not caused by conditions that, in the Navajo setting, result in extremes of hospital use.

These findings suggest that we may be observing a cohort effect. The group below 75 includes in its number a few people with diseases sufficiently severe that in all likelihood they will not survive beyond their late seventies (indeed several died in the follow-up period). It is possible that the older cohort has already experienced such a loss of members, and that those who remain are impaired in a variety of ways that make them dependent on help different from that provided in a general hospital.

It is, of course, possible that among the people who were not hospitalized are some as sick as those we found needing substantial levels of hospital care. To examine this possibility, we have scrutinized those people with PHYSIP scores in the 90th percentile who were not hospitalized. There were 11 people in this category, four below the age of 75 and seven, 75 and above. Of the former, three had osteoarthritis, two of whom also had diabetes and the third of whom had a crippled limb from what is presumed to have been childhood paralytic polio. The fourth person had Parkinson's disease. Among the people 75 and above were four people with severe osteoarthritis, two of whom were also senile. A fifth and sixth were each blind, deaf, and occasionally confused, and the seventh had very severe rheumatoid arthritis.

These data suggest that the people with extreme PHYSIP scores who were not hospitalized were not suffering from diseases like those that led to extensive hospital use. In essence, these people are no different from those with high PHYSIP scores who were hospitalized less than 40 days in the course of the 3.5 years 1980-1983.

We have already shown that Navajos are one of those populations in which the mortality crossover seems to occur. We have also suggested that in our own sample there appears to be a cohort effect in which the young-old include within their number a disproportionate share of people who are extensive users of hospital services. At the same time, however, our measure of physical functioning is correlated with age: older people report lower levels of function than do younger people.

To consider the issue of fitness more directly, we may compare our sample to a sample from a more affluent population with higher mortality at old age than the Navajos. For comparison we have chosen a sample of non-institutionalized elderly people studied by Katz et al. (1983) in Massachusetts. (See also Branch & Fowler, 1975; Branch, Katz, Kniepmann, & Papsidero, 1984). The two measures on which we have adequate data are dressing and transfer. Independence in dressing is defined as "gets clothes from closets and drawers; puts on clothes, outer garments, braces; manages fasteners; act of tying shoes is excluded." Independence in transfer is defined as "moves in and out of bed independently and moves in and out of chair independently (may or may not be using mechanical support)" (Katz & Akpom, 1976: 496). We have not included data on bathing since the situation for our informants is not comparable to that of people in Massachusetts in respect to the availability of facilities. Due to an oversight on out part, we did not include questions regarding eating, so no comparison is possible. Toileting and continence were not included in the Massachusetts data. Table 6.15 displays the results.

The differences between Navajos and people of the same age living in Massachusetts are not significant. Indeed, in their eighties Navajos tend to report slightly lower levels of independence. On the other hand, a higher proportion of the population 65 and above in Massachusetts is in extended care facilities than is true of Navajos, and it is thus possible that the non-institutionalized populations differ as a result. Rough

Table 6.15 Proportion at Each Age Who Are Independent

Age	Transferring		Dressing		
	Mass. %	Navajos %	Mass. %	Navajos %	Total No. Navajos
65-9	99.0	100.0	96.0	94.5	73
70-4	96.9	97.4	95.6	97.4	78
75-9	99.4	95.0	95.8	95.0	40
80-4	93.5	97.6	89.6	85.7	42
≥ 85	91.7	88.6	83.3	80.0	35

SOURCE: Branch and Fowler, 1975

calculations assuming (1) 3 percent utilization in Massachusetts (comparable to what we have estimated for the Navajos), and (2) that the Massachusetts people in our estimate now no longer institutionalized are all dependent in dressing and transfer, do not alter the results significantly, however. On the whole, we do not think the crossover phenomenon has resulted in surviving Navajos having dramatically better levels of function than people of the same age in the comparison population.

These results are congruent with those of a study of a nationwide sample of elderly Indians (60 years of age and above) compared with a sample of elderly (65 years of age and above) poor, non-Indian residents of Cleveland, Ohio. The Older Americans Resources and Services (OARS) instrument was used and provides more adequate comparative data than our survey did, though the age groups are not identical. If anything, however, the differences bias the results in such a way as to make the Indians look more like non-Indians than they probably are in fact. This is because the Indians in the survey were younger than the non-Indians.

In general, the results show that the Indian respondents consistently reported a higher level of disability than the non-Indians. For example, 2.2 percent of Indians as compared with 1.2 percent of non-Indians reported they were unable to walk; 1.4 percent of Indians and 0.8 percent of non-Indians were unable to get in and out of bed; 1.1 percent of Indians and 0.3 percent of non-Indians could not feed themselves; and 2.2 percent of Indians and 1.4 percent of non-Indians could not dress and undress themselves without help (National Indian Council on Aging, 1981, pp. 133-134).

SPECIFIC HEALTH CONDITIONS

We have had occasion to distinguish between measures of function and nosologic entitities. It is appropriate here to consider some of those specific conditions in more detail. We shall consider briefly accidents, alcohol abuse, and diabetes.

We have already observed that accidents among Navajos account for the greatest number of years of life lost of all causes of death, particularly among men; they continue to be a significant cause of death into old age; and they are far more significant as a cause of death among Navajos at all ages than they are among non-Indians. The three accidental deaths in our sample of elderly people were all men struck by motor vehicles as they walked along or crossed a road. There is a possibility that at least one of them was drunk at the time he was killed, but this is not certain. Thus, there is some suggestive evidence that elderly Navajos may be the victims of others' careless driving rather than themselves being the reckless drivers who cause accidents.

The conventional wisdom is that alcohol abuse is a major cause of accidents of all sorts. There is some evidence that this may indeed be the case, but it is not nearly as firm as one would like. In a study of fatal automobile accidents, Katz and May (1979) showed that alcohol was thought by the investigating officer to be involved in about as high a proportion of accidents among Navajos as among non-Navajos. But because accidents, particularly motor vehicle accidents, are so much more common among Navajos, the absolute contribution of alcohol is probably greater.

The pattern of alcohol use among Navajos has changed over the past 20 years, and there has been little detailed study of the phenomenon since our work in the late 1960s and early 1970s (Levy & Kunitz, 1974). Men and women have typically used alcohol very differently. It was not uncommon for men to drink heavily in binges separated by weeks or months, to experience withdrawal symptoms, and to diminish or cease alcohol consumption in their late thirties or early forties. Women generally tended to be abstainers, but when they did drink, it was often as a result of serious psychological difficulties. Women who drank to excess were much more likely to be social isolates than men who drank equally heavily.

In the 1960s, deaths from alcoholic cirrhosis occurred at lower rates among Navajos than among non-Indians. In the 1970s, the patterns changed. Among both men and women under 65, death rates from cirrhosis were higher among Navajos than non-Navajos. At age above 65, rates among Navajo women were higher than non-Indian rates whereas rates among Navajo men were lower (Kunitz, 1983, p. 104).

In our study of 271 elderly Navajo men and women we did not investigate alcohol use as thoroughly as in retrospect we should have. Two important findings do stand out, however. In a study of the prevalence of treated hypertension in this sample, we observed that there was no association between self-reported alcohol use and hyertension among men, but that among women there was an association. "For a considerable number of women we have no information regarding drinking patterns, and among the women from whom we do have information very few are currently drinking. But of the five who were reported to be still using alcohol at the time of the study, four had been diagnosed as hypertensive" (Kunitz & Levy, 1986, p. 110). These results were interpreted to be congruent with the results we had obtained in our previous studies: that few women drink but that those who do tend to have other problems as well. Of course as norms of behavior change, women's drinking behavior may have become much altered, particularly among young adults.

In a study of mortality and social isolation in this same sample, we observed that unmarried men were at greater risk of dying in the follow-up period than married men, and that among women there was no association between marital status and risk of mortality. Among the men, moreover, it was observed that unmarried men were particularly likely to live without their children or other kin, which is to say, they were the ones who were especially likely to be isolated. They were also the ones who were especially likely to be heavy drinkers. What was not clear from the interviews was whether drinking was a cause or a result of isolation in these men. Whatever the case, it seemed to put them at increased risk of dying in the three-year period of follow-up.

The third problem we shall discuss briefly is noninsulin dependent diabetes, a disease that has reached epidemic proportions in some American Indian tribes, particularly the Pimas in southern Arizona, for reasons that are as yet unclear but seem to be the result of both genetic factors and changes in diet and exercise patterns. Among Navajos, the fear is that the incidence and prevalence are both increasing. Such an increase seems likely but has not yet reached catastrophic proportions. In our sample of 271 elderly men and women, the prevalence of diabetes known to the health care system was 17 percent. Two deaths in our sample were due to renal failure secondary to diabetes. We do not have good data on other sequelae of the disease in this sample, but it is clear that there were a number of cases of diabetic retinopathy, peripheral neuropathy, and the like. It used to be the conventional wisdom that elderly Navajos could walk about with high blood sugar levels and not develop the sequelae of diabetes. That impression now seems to have been due to the fact that diabetes was being observed at the very beginning of the increases, before people had had it long enough to develop the sequelae. It is to be feared that the problem will become worse in future unless preventive measures are taken.

DISCUSSION

We have shown that Navajos have higher mortality than non-Indians at ages below 65, and lower mortality at ages above 65, particularly among women. This seems to be a pattern that is characteristic of all American Indians, not only Navajos (Markides, 1983).

It is of both theoretical and practical significance to know whether increased mortality at young ages is associated with the survival of healthier people into old age. Hospital utilization data suggest an affirmative response. Elderly Navajos have lower rates of utilization than non-Indians of the same age. On the other hand, the use of extended care facilities is not significantly different among Navajos and non-Navajos of the same age in Arizona and New Mexico. We believe that characteristics of the health care system probably determine these patterns. The limited availability of long-term beds in Arizona and New Mexico, both on and off the reservation, affects all elderly people about equally. And hospital utilization is low, we believe, not because elderly Navajos do not experience physical problems to the same degree as non-Indians, but because the kind of disability they experience is not considered appropriate for hospital admission.

We have suggested that there are two forms of morbidity that are distinguishable: (1) discrete nosological entities of greater or lesser severity that may or may not be reflected in measures of physical dysfunction; and (2) nonspecific functional problems that seem to be the consequences of aging itself.

Severe nosological entities associated with high levels of dysfunction (e.g., respiratory and renal failure) are found most commonly in people below the age of 75 who are likely to die by the time they reach their late seventies. More diffuse problems of physical and psychosocial dysfunction that increase in frequency and severity with advancing age may not be associated with life-threatening disease and may not themselves be life-threatening in an adequately protected environment.

Our findings suggest that Navajos may experience the first form of morbidity in their sixties and seventies, and this may reduce the proportion of people with life-threatening diseases at older ages. It does not seem to reduce the proportion of people who have problems in carrying out activities of daily living. Similar results are observed in a study of elderly Indians from a nationwide sample compared with a sample of non-Indian urban poor people. Thus, it is partly correct to say that some sort of winnowing process does occur. But it is not correct to assume that the survivors are, therefore, free of disease and, thus, not in need of a variety of supports, both professional and domestic, in order to continue to manage adequately.

REFERENCES

Aberle, D. F. (1981). A century of Navajo kinship change. *Canadian Journal of Anthropology, 2,* 21-36.

Bergner, M., Bobbitt, R. A., Kressel, S., Pollard, W. E., Gibson, B. S., & Morris, J. R. (1976a). The sickness impact profile: Conceptual formulation and methodology for the development of a health status measure. *International Journal of Health Services, 6,* 393-415.

Bergner, M., Bobbitt, R. A., Pollard, W. E., Martin, D. M., & Gibson, B. S. (1976b). The sickness impact profile: Validation of a health status measure. *Medical Care, 14,* 57-67.

Branch, L. G., & Fowler, F. J. (1975). *The health care needs of the elderly and chronically disabled in Massachusetts.* Boston: Survey Research Program of the University of Massachusetts and the Joint Center for Urban Studies of M.I.T. and Harvard University.

Branch, L. G., Katz, S., Kniepmann, K., & Papsidero, J. A. (1984). A prospective study of functional status among community elders. *American Journal of Public Health, 74,* 266-268.

Broudy, D. W., & May, P. A. (1983). Demographic and epidemiologic transition among the Navajo Indians. *Social Biology, 30,* 1-16.

Bureau of the Census. (1982). *Census of population and housing, 1980: Summary tape file 1.* Washington, DC: U.S. Department of Commerce.

Bureau of Indian Affairs. (1972). *Navajo population estimate. Office of Information and Statistics.* Window Rock, AZ: Navajo Area Office, Bureau of Indian Affairs, Department of the Interior.

Carr, B. A. (1978). *Projection of Navajo male and female elderly through the year 2000.* Window Rock, AZ: Department of Aging, Navajo Tribe.

Carr, B. A., & Lee, E. S. (1978). Navajo tribal mortality: A life table analysis of the leading causes of death. *Social Biology, 25,* 279-287.

Coale, A. J., & Kisker, E. E. (1986). Mortality crossovers: Reality or bad data? *Population Studies, 40,* 389-401.

Department of Health Services. (1977). *Sickness impact profile.* Seattle: School of Public Health, University of Washington.

Fulmer, H. S., & Roberts, R. W. (1963). Coronary heart disease among the Navajo Indians. *Annals of Internal Medicine, 59,* 740-764.

Gilson, B. S., Gilson, J. S., Bergner, M., Bobbitt, R. A., Kressel, S., Pollard, W. E., Vesselago, M. (1975). The sickness impact profile: Development of an outcome measure of health care. *American Journal of Public Health, 65,* 1304-1310.

Goodman, J. M. (1982) *The Navajo atlas: Environments, resources, people, and history of the Dine Bikeyah.* Norman: University of Oklahoma Press.

Henderson, E. B. (1979). Skilled and unskilled blue collar Navajo workers: Occupational diversity in an American Indian tribe. *The Social Science Journal, 16,* 63-80.

Johnston, D. F. (1966). An analysis of sources of information on the population of the Navajo (Bulletin 197, Bureau of American Ethnology). Washington, DC: U.S. Government Printing Office.

Katz, P. S., & May, P. A. (1979). *Motor vehicle accidents on the Navajo reservation, 1973-1975.* Window Rock, AZ: Navajo Health Authority.

Katz, S., & Akpom, C. A. (1976). A measure of primary sociobiological functions. *International Journal of Health Services, 6,* 493-508.

Katz, S., Branch, L. G., Branson, M. H., Papsidero, J. A., Beck, J. C., & Greer, D. S. (1983). Active life expectancy. *New England Journal of Medicine, 309,* 1218-1224.

Kelly, L. C. (1968). *The Navajo Indians and federal Indian policy.* Tucson: University of Arizona Press.

Kunitz, S. J. (1983). *Disease change and the role of medicine.* Berkeley and Los Angeles: University of California Press.

Kunitz, S. J., & Levy, J. E. (1986). The prevalence of hypertension among elderly Navajos: A test of the acculturative stress hypothesis. *Culture, Medicine and Psychiatry, 10,* 97-121.

Kunitz, S. J., & Slocumb, J. C. (1976). The changing sex ratio of the Navajo Tribe. *Social Biology, 23,* 33-44.

Levy, J. E. (1980). Who benefits from energy resource development: The special case of the Navajo Indians. *The Social Science Journal, 17,* 1-19.

Levy, J. E., & Kunitz, S. J. (1974). *Indian drinking: Navajo practices and Anglo-American theories.* New York: John Wiley.

Markides, K. S. (1983). Mortality among minority populations: A review of recent patterns and trends. *Public Health Reports, 98,* 252-260.

National Indian Council on Aging. (1981). *American Indian elderly: A national profile.* Albuquerque: National Indian Council on Aging.

National Master Facility Inventory (NMFI) (1983). *Nursing and related care homes as reported from the 1980 NMFI survey. National Heath Survey* (Series 14, No. 29 DHHS Publication No. (PHS) 84-1824). Hyattsville, MD: U.S. Department of Health and Human Services, Public Health Service, National Center for Health Statistics.

Navajo Tribe. (1978). *Navajo population estimates. Information Service Department.* Window Rock, AZ: Navajo Tribe.

Parman, D. L. (1976). *The Navajos and the new deal.* New Haven: Yale University Press.

Pollard, W. E., Bobbitt, R. A., Bergner, M., Martin, D. P., & Gilson, B. S. (1976). The sickness impact profile: Reliability of a health status measure. *Medical Care, 14,* 146-155.

Reno, P. (1981). *Mother Earth, Father Sky, and economic development: Navajo resources and their use.* Albuquerque: University of New Mexico Press.

U.S. Public Health Service. (1957). *Health services for American Indians.* (U.S. Department of Health, Education and Welfare, PHS Publication No. 531). Washington, DC: U.S. Government Printing Office.

Waldo, D. R., & Lazenby, H. C. (1984). Demographic characteristics and health care use and expenditures by the aged in the United States: 1977-1984. *Health Care Financing Review, 6,* 1-29.

Weatherby, N. L., Nam, C. B., & Isaac, L. W. (1983). Development, inequality, health care, and mortality at the older ages: A cross-national analysis. *Demography, 20,* 27-43.

Wing S., Manton, K. G., Stallard, E., Hames, C. G., & Tyroler, H. A. (1985). The black/white mortality crossover: Investigation in a community-based study. *Journal of Gerontology, 40,* 78-84.

Wood, J. J. (1980). Rural western Navajo household income strategies. *American Ethnologist, 7,* 493-503.

Index

ABOUT THE CONTRIBUTORS

JEANNINE COREIL, Ph.D., received her doctorate in applied social anthropology from the University of Kentucky in 1979. She is currently Associate Professor at the Department of Community and Family Health of the University of South Florida in Tampa. She has published extensively on ethnicity, culture, and health. Over the last ten years, she has directed a variety of research projects in Haiti, focusing on maternal and child health issues.

JULIE ANN GREEN, B.A., is a Research Associate at the University of Miami's Center on Adult Development and Aging. She received her B.A. in psychology at New College (Honors College of the University of South Florida). Her current research interests include critically evaluating diagnostic protocol for Alzheimer's patients, examining social service use by demented Hispanics and their caregivers, and catalyzing community outreach to "underprivileged" older adults.

JACQUELYNE JOHNSON JACKSON, Ph.D., is a pioneer in ethnogerontology. She received her doctorate in sociology from the Ohio State University in 1960. Her numerous publications since 1967 about social and related aspects of aging among blacks and other minorities include *Minorities and Aging* (1980). A member of the Duke University faculty since 1966, she has presented many invited lectures and addresses and conducted a number of workshops on ethnogerontology. A recipient of a number of awards for her professional work, she also holds membership in various professional organizations. The editor of the *Journal of Minority Aging,* a founder of the National Caucus on Black Aged in 1970, and the instigator of the National Center on Black Aged, she has helped to dispel unwarranted myths about American blacks.

STEPHEN J. KUNITZ, M.D., Ph.D., is Associate Professor at the Department of Preventive and Rehabilitation Medicine of the University of Rochester School of Medicine. In addition to his research among American Indians of the Southwest, he has done research in the history of medicine and the history of mortality.

JERROLD E. LEVY, Ph.D., is Professor at the Department of Anthropology of the University of Arizona. He has worked extensively among the Indians of the Southwest in the area of medical anthropology. He is currently a National Endowment for the Humanities Resident Scholar at the School of American Research in Santa Fe, New Mexico. His book on Navajo seizure disorders was published in 1988.

CHARLES F. LONGINO, Jr., Ph.D., is Professor of Sociology and Associate Director of the Center for Adult Development and Aging of the University of Miami. He received his doctorate in sociology from UNC-Chapel Hill and a post-doctorate from the Midwest Council for Social Research in Aging. His most widely reported research projects have used census microdata to profile understudied sectors of the older population; among these are the Retirement Migration Project, the Oldest Americans, and the Pension Elite Projects.

KYRIAKOS S. MARKIDES, Ph.D., received his doctorate in sociology from Louisiana State University in 1976. He is currently Professor in the Division of Sociomedical Sciences, Department of Preventive Medicine and Community Health, the University of Texas Medical Branch at Galveston. He has conducted extensive research on aging and health with special focus on the Mexican American population of the Southwest. Among his many publications is *Aging and Ethnicity* (coauthored with Charles H. Mindel, Sage, 1987). He is also the founding editor of the new *Journal of Aging and Health* (Sage).

LINDA PERKOWSKI ROGERS is a Ph.D. candidate in the Department of Preventive Medicine and Community Health of the University of Texas Medical Branch at Galveston. She is currently involved in analyzing data from the Hispanic Health and Nutrition Examination Survey, with focus on middle-aged and older people.

CHARLOTTE PERRY, M.P.H., received her degree from the University of North Carolina at Chapel Hill. She is the junior author who assisted Dr. Jackson in compiling the data for Chapter 4. A member of the North Carolina A. & T. State University faculty in Greensboro, Mrs. Perry, a registered nurse, is also a doctoral student in the Department of Child Development and Family Relations, School of Home Economics, University of North Carolina at Greensboro.

LOIS M. VERBRUGGE, Ph. D., received her doctorate in sociology from the University of Michigan in 1974. She is currently Associate Research Scientist at the Institute of Gerontology of the University of Michigan. She has numerous publications on the health of men and women, as well as on the health and health behavior of older people. She is now analyzing national data on the precursors of disability among persons with arthritis, and is conducting a longitudinal study on osteoarthritis and disability and their relation to physical and social activities.

GEORGE J. WARHEIT, Ph.D., is Professor and Chair of the Sociology Department and Professor of Psychiatry at the University of Miami. He received his doctorate from Ohio State University. His areas of interest are medical sociology, epidemiology, and comparative mental health studies. He was principal investigator of the NIAAA grant, "An Epidemiologic Study of Alcohol Use, Problem Drinking and Alcohol Dependence Among An Aging Population."